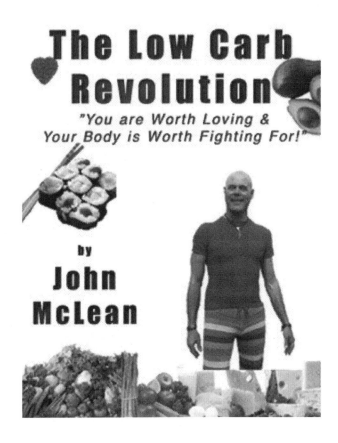

For my beautiful and brilliant daughter:
Oona McLean

The Low Carb Revolution by John McLean

"Things do not change...we change"
—Henry David Thoreau

Also by John McLean

*GET PUBLISHED NOW! The Step-by-Step Guide to
Writing & Publishing Your First Book on Amazon Kindle*

Introduction
"Welcome to the Revolution!"

Letting Go of the Past

Hi, thank you for joining the Revolution!

Thank you for taking a stand for yourself and for announcing to the world, "I will no longer fight against my Body. From now on I am fighting *for* it!" You're joining this revolution because *you* are worth it!

You deserve to feel good about yourself once again. You deserve to overflow with energy, vitality and health.

We've all made mistakes in the past. Yet that's why it's called the past, because it's behind us now. As of this moment you have your entire destiny directly ahead of you.

By taking time out of your busy schedule to read the *Low Carb Revolution* and learn more about how your Body and Mind function—how they *really* work together—you're sending an important message to yourself that says...

"Change is coming!"

Believe me, I know from long personal experience and from working with private clients over the years that change can be a little scary. Or even a lot scary! So I admire your courage and your willingness to let go of the missteps of the past.

I appreciate the boldness you've summoned from deep within to take this big step forward in your

4

pursuit of a triumphant return to your Ideal Body.

Your Ideal Body, of course, is the place where you feel most connected with your beautiful body.

It has nothing whatsoever to do somebody else's notion of how much you "should" weigh. You're not going to find your Ideal Body on a computer-generated chart or graph!

I recommend you pick an Ideal Body benchmark that you feel comfortable with that allows you to enjoy an active, healthy lifestyle. It doesn't even have to be a number.

Your "Ideal Body" can be a waist-size or a dress-size or even a *feeling*. A feeling in your body that lets you know, "This is it. My body has reached a sustainable shape and size where I feel that I can thrive!"

The Road Less Traveled

The path we're going to travel together in these pages definitely falls into the category of the road less traveled!

We're embarking on a unique adventure into body and mind completely unlike anything else you've ever experienced.

Along the way we're going to repeatedly rock any of our previous understandings of how we gain weight and why we gain it.

We'll challenge the very foundations of how we *thought* our brains worked, how we *believed* our habits were formed, and what we were *told* is even possible about making profound transformations in our lives.

As we do this, let's never forget the purpose of our Revolution! It's an impassioned protest against obesity, against feeling tired and sick all the time, and against the complacency and lethargy of those who all too often don't support us when we need it the most.

And it's a Revolution *for* something.

It's a Revolution for ourselves. For reclaiming our birthright of health, for returning to our natural state of our Ideal Body and Ideal Weight, as well as for realizing our worthiness to feel safe and loved.

We're creating this Revolution together because we are worth loving...and our bodies are worth fighting for!

Waking Up

So many people these days are simply frozen into inaction. They don't know what to do to improve their lives...and so they do nothing.

Even though their eyes seem to be open and they walk and talk and punch the clock at their jobs and spend every penny they earn (and then some!) at the mall every weekend, the majority of these teeming millions are, for all intents and purposes, *sleep-walking through life!*

You know who I'm talking about. You've seen these people. Maybe you've even seen them up close and personal?!

Now one of our principal goals here together, of course, is to discover the hidden mechanisms within the body that cause it to store and maintain fat.

By learning the actual physiology of weight gain and weight loss, we'll be able to make eating decisions from now on that can lead us to one of two outcomes...either to put on the pounds if we want, or let go of the pounds, if that's our deepest desire..

Another goal of ours will be to learn the *secrets* behind how our minds work and how our habits — the good, the bad and the ugly — are formed.

This will benefit us not just in making changes to our weight and overall lifestyle, but also give us the strength and the confidence to let go of any other negative patterns that we no longer desire.

6

But perhaps our most important goal of all is what I refer to as waking ourselves up.

Only when we finally wake up and *get here* can we devote ourselves to expressing our true, innermost passions in the world.

We're going to do all this—and more…much, much more!—in a space where at all times we can feel safe and loved.

"I have decided to stick with love. Hate is too great a burden to bear."
— Martin Luther King

Feeling Protected

For change to naturally emerge from within us, we all need the strong arms of safety and love to be wrapped tightly around us, day and night. And that's why I created the Low Carb Revolution audio affirmations that are included at no charge with your copy of this book..

You can access these affirmations online and download them instantly for FREE by visiting this address:

http://db.tt/69WOj7pW

You can also use this alternate download site in the event that the DropBox account above is moving slower than a groundhog in a marshmallow bog…

http://www15.zippyshare.com/v/36838740/file.html

These positive affirmations deliver a 30-minute dose

of encouragement, love, safety and support for your journey.

Don't just listen to them once, or even just once a day. Play them steadily in the background as much as possible while you read this book and go about the other activities of your busy life.

These audio affirmations were carefully designed to become your daily companion, travel partner and virtual bodyguard on the beautiful journey you have bravely undertaken.

The mp3 recording located at the address above provides helpful reiterations of many of the important secrets and techniques that you'll discover in this book.

The affirmations also contain supportive reminders of why you're undertaking this journey for yourself.

Finally, the affirmations contain the loving encouragement we *all* need to step outside our comfort zones and embrace a whole new world of adventure, excitement and possibility as we take a trip that ultimately leads us to the amazing destination called our Ideal Body.

The audio affirmations are double-tracked, with parallel messages aimed at the left and the right hemispheres of the brain playing in tandem.

Play them often. The more you play them in the background, the more supported and the more confident you will feel with each bold new step we take together.

And, unlike a traditional audio book or podcast, you don't even have to focus and listen to them with your full attention.

Simply play the affirmations in the background at a low level—where you almost have to strain to hear them—and the important reminders of love and support, as well as the summaries of the best practices in changing your eating and living habits to let go of any excess weight, will sink down into every cell of your body.

Once your cells finally understand what you really want and need from them, you'll have a Tribe of 65 trillion members working together to create magic in your life, in your body and in the world as a whole.

It really is that simple...and it really is that beautiful. Thank you again for playing!

"Two roads diverged in a wood, and I...I took the one less traveled by, and that has made all the difference."
—Robert Frost

The Low Carb Revolution
An Inner Journey and an Outer Journey

A Tale of Two Journeys

The revolutionary journey we're going on together in this book actually takes place in two different dimensions.

The first dimension is the *physical* one, if you will, where we concern ourselves with why we gain weight and what to eat in order to lose that weight and all sorts of little-known, science-y stuff about the physiology of how our bodies work.

The second dimension deals with the unseen inner world of our *brains*. We'll shine a bright light into this place of former mystery and misunderstanding as we discover why we make the choices we make, how we fall into the ruts of our various habits, and methods to pull ourselves back out again.

Only by exploring both of these equally important dimensions — one outside of us (the food we put in our bodies) and the other within us (our wounds, our fears, our habits and our negative thoughts) — can we succeed in our bold revolution of reclaiming our health and waking up to who we are and why we're really here.

The fatal flaw in most old-fashioned diets is they completely overlook the internal "front" in our heads where our own personal 'Battle of the Bulge' must also be waged.

Look, if JUST changing the way we eat was all it

took to lose weight, then pretty much *any* diet should be successful...instead of pretty much *none* of them, right?!

The First Dimension of our Journey

In Part One of the *Low Carb Revolution* we're going to jump in with both feet!

In a series of **13 Keys**, we will learn the exact mechanisms for how the storage of fats in our bodies is triggered...and what we can do to stop storing new fat and begin burning away the old fat we'd previously put away.

This will be followed by **13 Progressions**, where we'll discover the specific types of food and drink to consume (or to avoid) in order to effectively and permanently lose all the weight we've ever desired. Best of all, we'll do this with...

Absolutely NO calorie-counting or portion control.

Joining the *Low Carb Revolution* means you'll be able to eat as much as you like, as often as you like, every single day of the week and still lose weight!

Look, you already know that restricted-calorie diets and draconian portion controls not only don't work but also leave you feeling miserable, unsatisfied and unhappy.

And the more you deprive yourself of food, the less energy and vitality you have to contribute anything meaningful to the rest of the human race.

One of our goals here together is to help you feel exactly the *opposite* of miserable, unsatisfied and unhappy.

And another is to help you reclaim the energy and vitality that are necessary to accomplish your dreams and live the fulfilled, successful life you so richly desire and deserve.

So Part One covers the eating portion of our program, but that's just the very start of our adventure together.

The Second Dimension of our Journey

In Part Two we'll go even deeper.

In the **13 Secrets** that make up the second half of this book, I guarantee you'll learn more about yourself and why you do the things you do, as well as how your habits are formed and how to change them, then you previously learned in your whole entire life up until now!

A bold claim, I know! But the theories and models and metaphors of how we really operate from the inside out that I'll be sharing with you are *nothing* like anything you've ever been exposed to before, I promise you!

The strategies and techniques you will learn truly are that unique and, well, revolutionary! And not just revolutionary, but *necessary*.

Because if we can't effectively and permanently change our *habits*, then we won't be able to change the way we eat. And if we can't change the way we eat, we can't change how much we weigh. But even more importantly, without knowing how to change our habits from the inside out, we won't ever be able to fundamentally change who we are now and—who we can become! The self-proclaimed "Diet Gurus" somehow always leave out this rather significant step when dispensing their dieting advice!

Losing Weight is About Changing *You*

How many times has a diet guru told you, "I know you've been eating dessert after dinner each night for the last 30 years, but this is a dessert-free diet, so don't do that anymore." And in very next sentence, they go on to tell you the next huge, life-long habit you're supposed to instantly and magically change about yourself.

Well, habits are not quite that easy to change — that's *why* they're called habits.

That is to say, habits are not easy to change until you know HOW to change them, in the same way that French is quite difficult to speak until you learn *how* to speak French...and then speaking it becomes something you can do without even thinking about it.

As "monumental" as finally learning the secret to changing your own habits may appear, this is just a small portion of the personal transformation we'll be undergoing in Part Two of the *Low Carb Revolution*.

Now if you only read Part One of this book — and just learn about the mechanisms of how we create and store fat, as well as what foods to eat and which to avoid in order to create and store *less* of it — then you can and you will lose weight.

But this is a revolution here, so why should we stop there?!

You and I are not going through this entire experience together *only* to change how much you weigh! Yes, that's a big part of it, but there's another reason our paths have crossed at this particular juncture in your life...not sooner, and not later.

We've been brought together right now to change YOU!

Here's a crucial understanding I want to share with you right up front, and it's one we will return to again and again...

Losing Weight isn't just about changing what you eat... it's also about changing Who you Are!

So many people in the world spend their entire lives

blundering along, not sure what they're supposed to be doing, not sure where they're going and never finding out why they're even *here*!

If you read the entirety of the *Low Carb Revolution* and listen to the accompanying audio affirmations, you *will* open yourself up to a profoundly original understanding of who you are and Why You Are Here — perhaps for the first time ever.

"Some drink deeply from the river of knowledge. Others only gargle."
—Woody Allen

The Era of the "Diet Gurus" is Over

Frankly, we've been misled by many of the self-appointed Diet Gurus. And mislead really is the best word for it.

It's not like they don't want to help guide you on this journey of a lifetime...it's just they don't have a functional map, so they don't know which direction to point you.

Most of them are well-intentioned. Most of them secretly wish they could create a working map to teach good people just like yourselves how to lose weight and transform themselves.

I personally believe that when diet gurus lay their heads on their pillows every night they're just as scared as their followers.

Actually, they're probably even *more* scared, because they *know* they're just wandering along blindly, hoping to stumble upon the secret to how our minds and our bodies work together — or, more often, work against one another.

And it's not just the diet pundits, it's the entire *50 BILLION dollar a year diet industry*.

I refer to it as Big Diet, because it has become just as

14

much a pervasive and permanent part of our world as Big Food, Big Pharmacy or Big Tobacco.

As we shall soon reveal, the divide between Big Food and Big Diet is no kind of divide at all. The very *same* multinational food corporations whose entire business model is built around fattening us up with low-cost sugars and carbohydrates masquerading as food are the very *same* corporations who OWN and/or exclusively DISTRIBUTE the "weight-loss" products of the so-called Diet Industry.

The people behind Big Diet spend their days caught up in the "busy-work" of splashy marketing, celebrity endorsements and colorful calorie-counting charts even as they preach the much the same, demonstrably false theory that the only way for us to lose weight is by eating fewer calories through will power and self-control.

> *"Webb [1980] tabulated a number of overeating studies and accurately determined that energy intake [calories] is not sufficient to predict weight gain or loss in any individual. Nevertheless, the caloric theory is widely accepted and has become deeply ingrained in the public psyche."*
> —Leighton Steward, Sam Andrews, MD, Morrison Bethea, MD & Luis Balart, MD in *SUGAR BUSTERS!*

Big Diet versus "Human Machines"

Big Diet sees us as merely human machines.

What they're selling us is the notion that we are automatons made of flesh…put few enough calories in one end and a perfect human body comes off the assembly line at the other end.

They fail to realize that our actions are influenced by what goes on deep within us, not by something we read on a glossy handout!

We are constantly being guided by our feelings and our wounds and our fears, not by the numbers on a scale.

In their defense, the people behind Big Diet never had the opportunity to sit down and make an intense, dedicated study in how we actually make the complicated decisions and choices in our life from moment to moment.

As you'll discover when I share my story during Part Two, I'm fortunate enough to have gone on a long, solitary journey involving many lonely years of study and discovery in my own life in order to return to share with you some profound secrets of weight loss and personal transformation in these pages.

Actually, a better way of putting it is to say I'll be "reminding" you of my discoveries.

Because I have a strong feeling you already know these secrets, deep within you, in a place you just can't quite put your finger on.

Again, the first big "secret" of losing weight I want to share with you is this…

Losing Weight isn't just about changing what you eat…it's also about changing Who you Are!

How do we accomplish that? How do we change Who we Are?!

For starters, by reading this entire book. Not just Part One and not just Part Two, but by discovering both the inner and the outer maps to our future success.

And by listening to the accompanying Audio Affirmations. And by changing the way we eat and the way we live according to the truths we discover here.

Let The Healing Begin

Just do these things, and you *will* become a different

person than you are now.

Coincidentally, you will also weigh less. And you will gain something else that's profoundly important to the specific journey you are on.

Which leads us to the second secret to losing weight that Big Diet hasn't told you because, frankly, they don't even know it...

Losing Weight is about healing...from the inside out.

In Part One, we're going to begin the process of *physically* healing our bodies by learning how to eat in a way that truly serves us and helps us return to our birthright and natural state of our Ideal Body.

In Part Two, we're going to initiate the process of *emotionally* healing ourselves and exploring places within us where we can at last forgive ourselves fully and love ourselves completely.

If that's a journey you're ready to take with me now, then we've found each other at exactly the right moment. Take my hand, if you will, and let's start down this picturesque path that leads directly to a beautiful new YOU!

Because the truth is that *you* are the most breathtaking destination ever created!

And I want to be there for you every step of the way. So, to up the ante, I'd like to offer you the ability to contact me *directly* at any time of day or night with your concerns, questions, feedback, suggestions, success stories or ideas about how you plan to change the world (hopefully for the better, but we'll take what we can get!). To do that I'm going to give you my *private email address.*

This email addy goes directly to my personal email account and not to some Timothy Ferriss-esque 4-Hour

Workweek cubicle gulag in the Philippines where some minions making 17.5 cents a day are answering my mail for me! No, this email address comes to me and only me.

Here it is: **zombiejohn@gmail.com**

I want to hear from you. I want to know what you think, what you feel and how you're doing. I want you to succeed on this journey of healing yourself and falling back in love with yourself, and if there's anything else I can do to help you, I want to be there for you.

All I ask in return is that *you* continue to be there for yourself, that you never give up on yourself and your beautiful dreams!

> *"The true profession of man is*
> *finding his way to himself."*
> —Hermann Hesse

It's Krap Time!

Okay, if you are currently overweight, now is the perfect time to have yourself some processed, sugarized, food-shaped chemicals. Or what I like to refer to as Krap!

Krap includes any "food" that has no resemblance to actual Food. Examples of Krap are Pringles, Goldfish (not the actual, swimming-around kind!), Cheese Whiz and PopTarts.

If you bought it off a Dollar Menu, it's Krap. If the first (and, often, second, third and fourth) ingredient in your "food" is some derivative of corn or sugar or wheat, it's Krap.

Indeed, if the thing you're eating has more than five ingredients, it's probably Krap. If it doesn't mold, rot or decompose on its own, it's Krap. If it contains so many chemicals that the manufacturers have to "enrich" it to give it the slightest nutritional value, it's Krap.

I think you get the idea! Hey, believe me, I get that Krap is yummy. And salty. And crunchy. And cheap.

But Krap is still a significant reason why Americans are so heavy and so unhealthy and why our mortality rate is now going in the *wrong direction* for the first time in this country's history.

Even so, the real point I'm making here is this: if you want to continue snacking on Krap while you begin reading Part One of the *Low Carb Revolution*, by all means do so. Listen to me now—this is important.

Trying to "cut back" or deny yourself Krap before you finally make the decision to change your current habits is counter-productive. Denying yourself Krap on a part-time basis while still living a Fat Food Lifestyle on a full-time basis sends the exact wrong message to your mind and body.

It sends a message that Krap is *precious*. It sends a message that if you just deny yourself long enough—an hour here or an hour there—then you can have some more Krap as a reward.

Listen, Krap is NOT precious. Krap—no matter how super-sized and super-sugarized it may be—is NOT a reward for anything. Krap is NOT your friend.

And since there's nothing precious or rewarding about Krap, there's absolutely no reason for us to put off having any of it...until we learn exactly what it's been doing to our body and how it contributes to our waistline in ways we never prviously suspected. Does that make sense? Good! So now let's do it to it! Buckle your seat-belt, baby, grab a Twinkie and enjoy the ride!

"Bad things are not the worst things that can happen to us.
Nothing is the worst thing that can happen to us."
—Richard Bach

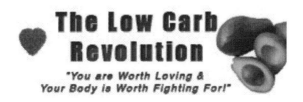

The Low Carb Revolution

*"You are Worth Loving &
Your Body is Worth Fighting For!"*

Part One:
"Why We Get Fat"

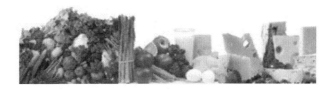

(NOTE: I am not a doctor, nor have I ever played one on TV! Any dietary advice or recommendations contained in this book should be considered as merely good suggestions that you should certainly run by your family doctor or physician and find out what they feel is best for you, especially if you have an ongoing illness or suspect you may be pregnant. Even if you're in the best of health and are only looking to drop a few pounds, always consult a licensed medical professional before embarking on any dietary changes.)

"You are the hero of your own story."
— Mary McCarthy

KEY #1:
"Being First is Always the Hardest"

The Remarkable Mr. Banting

Meet William Banting of 27 St. James's Street, Piccadilly, London. An undertaker by profession, Mr. Banting is a distinguished Englishman who has a wee bit of a problem.

He is — how shall we phrase it? — heavyset. Publicly, he admits to being corpulent; privately, he thinks of himself as fat. He's certainly aware of the jeers and sneers of his fellows regarding the more than 200 pounds he carries on his modest 5'5" frame.

William Banting desperately desires to lose weight, but he's already failed with every diet ever invented.

There's no fad, no quackery, no blatant hucksterism that's above his purchase. And his excess weight is not for lack of burning calories. In addition to the constant daily activity of being a busy undertaker, Mr. Banting goes for long walks, spends hours each morning rowing his own boat upon the Thames River that runs through the heart of London, and experiments with numerous other ways to exert himself enough to lose some pounds.

By his own account: "Few men have led a more active life."

Yet all his arduous exercise simply builds up muscle mass and makes him hungrier still...and in the end William Banting weighs even *more* than when he started his ambitious exercise program.

The physicians that Banting consults deduce he must still be taking in too many calories and so they sternly advise him to eat even less than his already meager daily intake of food.

The undertaker dutifully reduces his diet day by day until, finally, it's almost negligible. A man on a hunger strike could scarcely eat less.

Mr. Banting is consuming practically nothing…tea with cream and a few ticks of toast topped with butter and jam, yet he still isn't losing any weight and he feels listless and grumpy all the time — an experience that virtually all of us have also suffered through, I should imagine!

Out of desperation he finally consults a distinguished London Ear, Nose & Throat surgeon named Dr. William Harvey — no relation, by the way, to the more famous Dr. William Harvey who was a contemporary of Shakespeare and was the first person to accurately describe the circulation of blood within humans, a discovery that itself will play a dramatic role in the tale to come!

By sheer good fortune, this particular Dr. Harvey is fresh from attending a series of ground-breaking lectures in Paris on the causes of diabetes and its relationship to obesity, so the doctor possesses a rather advanced understanding of how the human body gains weight and even has a novel, untested idea for a mechanism by which weight can also be lost.

At Mr. Banting's earnest request, Dr. Harvey cobbles together an eating plan according to these revolutionary new principles of weight gain and loss.

The innovative diet suggested by the doctor allows Mr. Banting to eat and drink (including coffee, tea and a modest quantity of alcohol) in abundance, while simply avoiding what Banting refers to as "beans".

Avoiding "Beans"

Now these aren't literally beans, but rather Banting's clever moniker for the "forbidden" types of food that cause us to gain weight.

Banting lumps the few "bad foods" forbidden by Dr. Harvey together under the category of "beans".

So, to recap: The only thing Mr. Banting does differently on his new regime is to eat and drink a-plenty, while avoiding the so-called "beans"--the fat-causing foods and drinks. Beyond this, he does no extra exercise and takes no special tonics.

In his own droll, English fashion, William Banting describes the profound and utterly delightful changes in his body (and, indeed, his entire life) using the strategy of merely avoiding "beans"...

"Am reduced nearly 13 inches in bulk, and 50 lbs. in weight.
Can perform every necessary office for myself.
My sight and hearing are surprising at my age.
My other bodily ailments have become mere matters of history."
From the "Letter On Corpulence" by William Banting

A Happy Ending

In the space of less than a year, Mr. Banting lost a full fifty lbs. and kept these undesired pounds off for the rest of his long and productive life.

He enjoyed his remaining years in good health and vitality...even allowing himself to indulge in "beans" from time to time!

William Banting later encountered some notoriety by self-publishing his weight-loss story as the "Letter on Corpulence", which inspired legions of English men and women to follow in his footsteps and create success stories of their own by simply avoiding "beans"!

In fact, the weight-loss example of William Banting touched the popular imagination so deeply that the term "banting" is used interchangeably with "slimming" in England to this very day.

Almost by sheer happenstance, William Banting (or, more precisely, the good Dr. Harvey; no, not the famous one, the *other* one!) stumbled upon the ideal eating strategy for losing weight.

What makes this entire story even more remarkable is that neither man truly grasped the importance of their discovery...in large part because neither fully understood the physiology or the biochemistry behind it.

And that was because *nobody in the entire world* understood the science behind weight loss or weight gain (or most of the other complicated processes that take place within the human body) since Mr. Banting's delightful weight-loss story took place way back in eighteen-hundred and sixty-two!

So fully *150 years ago*, long before even our great-grandparents were born, the *secret* of how our body stores fat and releases fat was known...or at least strongly suspected!

Another Remarkable Mr. Banting

In the kind of ironic coincidence that can only happen in the real world, the man who ultimately helped explain the science behind William Banting's weight loss in 1862 was his direct relation, Dr. Frederick Banting, who won the Nobel Prize in 1923 as the co-discoverer of the hormone known as Insulin. A hormone, I should add, that will play a leading role in the drama unfolding before us.

Because it is the *relationship* between the "beans" of William Banting and the Insulin of his descendent Frederick Banting that forms the foundation of the remarkable "new" eating strategy you will be exposed to in Part One of the *Low Carb Revolution*.

So how's that for Breaking News?!

The principles behind the only eating plan ever discovered that successfully allows us to lose weight without portion controls, without counting calories and without beating ourselves up for lack of will-power or self-control have been known and available for our use for a good 150 years and counting!

And the science behind WHY eliminating "beans" from our diet leads directly to losing our unsightly belly fat has been understood for close to a century.

Even so, the vast majority of the human population today remains utterly unaware of either William Banting or Frederick Banting, and they remain unaware that by simply avoiding "beans" they can turn the tragedy of their weight-loss story into an outright comedy with a happy ending of its own.

In July 1956, G.L.S. Pawan, MD and Alan Kekwick, PhD published the results of a scientific evaluation of Banting's diet in the prestigious English medical journal, *Lancet*, proving that Banting and Harvey were right.

Here is their conclusion: "The composition of the diet can alter the expenditure of calories in obese persons, increasing it when fat and proteins are given, and decreasing it when carbohydrates are given."

The carbohydrates referred to here are, of course, William Banting's "beans".

From William Banting to your humble narrator—and with many tens of thousands of success stories in between—the principles you'll learn in the Low Carb Revolution have made it possible for ordinary people just like you and me to make a triumphant return to our birthright and natural state of our Ideal Body.

The Low Carb Revolution by John McLean

*"The very best proof that
something can be done is that
someone has already done it."*
--Bertrand Russell

KEY #2:
"We've Been Fighting the Wrong Enemy"

You Are Not to Blame

In the *Low Carb Revolution*, I'm going to make a strong case that YOU are not the enemy!

Despite what physicians, nutritionists and Big Diet have been beating you over the head with for decades now, this revolution is *not* against your supposed lack of self-control, weak will-power, laziness, or any of the other snide, disparaging terms they come up with such ease and regularity.

Quite the contrary!

What's amazing to me is the progress you've already made on your own, the successes you've managed to carve out in your life even before having a thorough understanding of how your body makes and stores fat.

I'm so impressed that you are here. I'm proud of you for taking this big step in fighting for your body. And I admire your courage in going on this journey with me.

Although many wonderful changes are in store for you just ahead, I want you to know that you are beautiful and loveable and perfect just the way you are right now!

I want to offer you another secret to losing weight that Big Diet hasn't told you—and never will, because this secret can't be manufactured into a pill, or processed into a powder or shake that they can sell you!

This secret includes a built-in goal. A goal that at first blush might seem difficult, if not impossible, to attain. Even *contemplating* this goal could make some people feel uncomfortable.

But I'm here to tell you that reaching this goal is the critical element that's been missing from almost every other weight-loss program most of us have failed at in the past.

Are you ready for the next secret? Here it is...

Losing weight is about falling in love with yourself... all over again!

Let that sink in for a moment, if you will. Feel in your body, right now, what that statement really *means*. Imagine what it would feel like to completely and totally love your body, exactly the way it is right now. (Hey, I warned you this secret might make you feel a little uncomfortable!)

> "If we really love ourselves, everything in
> our life works"
> —Louise Hay

Losing Weight is a Love Story

Losing weight is first, last, and always a Love Story. A love story about you.

If you'll stay with me on this journey the whole way through to the end of the book, you'll discover that loving yourself once again is not only possible but unavoidable.

I want you to fall in love with yourself...with who you are right now, as well as who you might become as a result of our work together.

I especially want you to fall in love with your

beautiful body...just as it is at this very moment.

When you truly accept and love and forgive every cell in the body you currently have, at the weight you currently weigh, only then can the healing begin.

Only then will your incredible body respond, and finally start making any and all of the dramatic changes you've desired for so long.

I also want you to fall in love with your Inner Self...that patiently waiting, shiny, glowy, amazing, powerful, loving and healing part of you that's been asleep deep within you all these years!

An All-New You!

Our admittedly ambitious goal here is nothing less than creating an all-new *you*!

In Part One you're going to discover how to feed yourself from the outside-in...and in Part Two, you'll learn how to love yourself from the inside-out!

Armed with this passionate new relationship with ourselves, as well as some profound strategies on how best to fuel our beautiful bodies, by the end of this quest we'll be well-prepared to head out into the big scary world of calories and processed sugars and laboratory-manufactured Krap...just like seasoned, battle-trained revolutionaries!

> *"Love yourself first and everything else falls in line. You really have to love yourself to get anything done in this world!"*
> — Lucille Ball

The Real Business at Hand

Once you've gone through both parts of the Low Carb Revolution, absorbed the learnings into your life and are moving in the direction of reconnecting with your incredible body once more, you will at last have the breathing room to focus on some of the other important things you desire from your life.

With your body "handled", you can look forward to spending time doing one of the most significant tasks that you've probably been neglecting for ages: being Amazing!

Listen, there's *nobody* like you in all the world. You are here for a reason. A unique, singular and important reason. And that reason is NOT to lose weight! If anything, the excess weight has just been holding you back from fulfilling your true potential.

We could even say the weight was just a place to hide from the world. Here's another essential secret to weight loss for you to process and incorporate into your life...

Losing weight is about no longer hiding...from yourself or from the world.

If you've ever been overweight, then you surely don't need me to explain this one. You know *exactly* what I'm talking about when I mention "hiding from the world," don't you?!

I know, I've been there!

When we become heavy, we're able to hide from the world and hide from ourselves, right in plain sight.

You might even say we *Insulin-ate* ourselves from having to deal with the problems around us!

The extra weight gave us something to hide behind. As the weight goes away, that leaves us a little more exposed and out in the open.

But, guess what? That's okay — by the time we get there, we'll be able to handle it!

That's what Part Two of this book was specifically written for, to help you through these awkward and inevitable feelings. And that's why you've been given the powerful audio affirmations as my special gift to you.

The audio affirmations will support you every step of the way if you'll just take advantage of them and play them in the background as often as possible.

Are you are ready to let your light shine brighter in the world than ever before?! Are you ready to do your dance, whatever it is?! Then let's stop hiding and go deeper!

> *"I don't like myself, I'm crazy*
> *about myself!"*
> —Mae West

KEY #3:
"There's Lies...and There's Damned Lies"

The Obesity Epidemic

No matter what your age, you probably grew up hearing over and over again about the plight of people starving to death throughout the developing world...and sometimes just around the corner from us in even in the most modern societies.

We were told that helping to end the hunger epidemic was one of the most significant contributions we could make in our lives.

And that remains true to this very day. Hunger continues to be a crushing problem in the world and any way we can help ameliorate it is a blessing.

At the same time, however, another epidemic has progressively insinuated itself in the fabric of our world—an epidemic with dire health implications and perhaps even less hope for immediate improvement.

Here's a sobering story that didn't exactly make yesterday's evening news...

In our lifetimes, the number of *over-nourished* people in the world has now far surpassed the number of under-nourished people. As of 2011, the World Heath Organization (WHO) estimated there are some 925 million people in the world who don't get enough to eat on a regular basis. That's a lot of hungry people.

At the same time, WHO projects we are already closing in on **2 billion** (that's BILLION with a "b"!)

overweight humans. And another 500 million are expected to join the ranks of the overweight within the next few years alone.

By the year 2015 an estimated 2.5 billion people in the world will be overweight!

Where did all these overweight people come from? Is everybody really stuffing their faces so full of calories and moving so little every day that they can't help but gain all this weight?!

Why is it the more that politicians and governments and committees get involved in providing "helpful" guidelines to educate their citizens about better eating choices, the *bigger* their citizens become?!

Seriously, what are all these overweight people doing so wrong that's causing this unprecedented explosion of heaviness in the human race?!

Lucky for you and me, we're going to learn the answers to these questions and more right here in Part One of the *Low Carb Revolution*.

But here's the answer in a nutshell: The reason we've become so overweight is that nobody ever sat us down and accurately described the *known mechanisms* of why we get fat and the specific steps we can take to *lose that fat*.

Before we discover the truths behind the solution to our global obesity nightmare, first let's touch briefly on what's *not* to blame for our ever-expanding waistlines.

> *"People are fed by the food industry,*
> *which pays no attention to health…and*
> *are treated by the health industry, which*
> *pays no attention to food."*
> —Wendell Berry

What's NOT Causing The Obesity Epidemic

Let's hijack Mark Twain's famous phrase, "There are lies and then there are damned lies." Over and over again we have been told four *damned lies* about losing weight. These are lies that are neither useful to us nor are they true.

These are lies that cause us to *gain* weight rather than lose weight. Lies that make us miserable where we should be happy. Lies that we're going to need to let go of so we can transform ourselves into revolutionaries fighting for the right of our bodies to be free and whole once again.

We have been told four particular lies about why we gain weight so often and so consistently that they have become part of the fabric of our culture. Despite all that, they remain not just lies, but Damned Lies!

"The 4 Damned Lies of Why We Are Overweight"

We are overweight because we eat too many calories

We are overweight because we don't burn enough calories

We are overweight because we eat fat

We are overweight because we have faulty genes

These damned lies are at the very heart of our global obesity nightmare, so let's touch on each of them in turn.

Lie #1: We're Overweight Because We Eat Too Many Calories

The truth is: *Calories alone don't make us fat.*

Yes, yes, yes, I realize the above statement is a heresy almost as unpardonable as Galileo's insistence that the earth revolves around the sun, rather than the other way around as had been taught since the beginning of civilization.

To this very day we are routinely informed by teachers, politicians and, especially, by the media that it's all about how much we eat.

If we eat too many calories, so the story goes, then we gain weight...and the only practical way to lose weight is to eat less of them.

But it wasn't always this way. Just a couple of short generations ago, most people didn't worry about calories at all...and they weren't growing particularly fat from eating too many of them. Thanks to cable TV and the Internet, it's now possible to time-travel back to the 1980's.

You don't need a Delorean with a banana-peel-fueled flux capacitor, all you gotta do is sit down in front of your computer or TV and watch some music videos from the earliest days of MTV.

Pick a band, any band, any artist, it doesn't matter. After watching a dozen or so classic music videos from the '80s, you'll be struck by something similar about every one of them. Everybody was almost annoyingly slim back then. The younger artists, the older artists, male, female, black, white, didn't seem to matter—almost everybody was thin.

Next check out some of the popular TV shows and motion pictures from the eighties. Same thing. Slim was in.

Yet nobody counted calories and certainly nobody paid any attention to fat.

Then something happened that changed everything. A new dietary craze emerged that led directly to where we are in the United States today—not only the fattest nation in the world, but the fattest nation in the history of the world!

The low-fat, low-calorie craze of the late '80s and early '90s told us to make our dietary choices *exclusively* on the calorie count of our foods, with a particular emphasis on eating more *carbohydrates* than ever before.

Although most people were not particularly overweight back then, we were told that the less fat and the fewer calories we ate, the better off we would be.

And so we complied. I mean, why wouldn't we? As we shall soon learn, the US government itself put its entire weight (so to speak!) behind these new dietary guidelines.

Yet since the low-fat/low-calorie fad began in the eighties, our collective weight has *exploded*. Every measurable category of weight-gain and worsening health has gone straight through the roof—the percentage of overweight people, the numbers of obese, the incidence of diabetes, and on and on.

Despite what we were led to believe, not only did the Low-Calorie Fad *not* work, but it made us all sicker and more overweight than ever before.

> *"The tiresome business of*
> *totting up daily calories, on*
> *which most modern reducing*
> *diets are based, is a waste of*
> *time for an obese person.*
> *Because, as Prof. Kekwick and*
> *Dr. Pawan showed, a fat man*
> *may maintain his weight on a*
> *low-calorie diet."*
> —Richard Mackarness, MD

1 Lb. Does NOT Equal 3500 Calories!

You already know to the depth of your being that restricted-calorie diets and portion-controls don't work. One of the reasons you know this is because you've probably tried calorie-counting in a desperate attempt to lose weight and you've failed at it—again and again and again.

Following the official guidelines of government agencies, you've cut much of the fat out of your diet, reduced calories, left food on your plate, eaten barely enough food to even sustain life...and done this day upon miserable day for week after depressing week. And then after months of suffering you discover you've lost 2 whole lbs or, more often, gained 3 new pounds!

Not only has the low-fat, calorie-counting fad *not* worked, it has made us fatter than ever before. You and every human alive who has ever "dieted" already knows this to your core.

The very first diet in recorded history, way back in Ancient Greece, involved a restricted calorie regime.

It didn't work 2500 years ago and it doesn't work today and that's not ever going to change.

Limiting our portions or counting the calories is not a realistic, practical, sustainable or scientific way to lose weight.

And yet the party-line of glossy magazines, calorie-counting weight-loss programs and card-carrying nutritionists remains that a pound of fat equals approximately 3500 calories.

We are told again and again that in order to lose a pound of fat, we "simply" have to create a *deficit* of 3500 calories and that pound of fat will magically disappear.

Of course, a pound does NOT equal 3500 calories and creating that deficit won't magically make it disappear, but let's play along for a moment and *pretend* that we live in a world where science and the laws of physics no longer apply.

The most popular restricted-calorie diet today aims to create a daily deficit of 1000 calories in their victims, errr, I mean clients.

So instead of a reasonable intake of, say, 2500 calories of food per day, the dieter is restricted to no more than 1500 calories.

Okay, let's put on our Pretend Caps and imagine this is actually an effective weight-loss strategy and do some math...

1000 calorie deficit per day x 7 days in a week = 7000 fewer calories not consumed over the course of the week.

Therefore, 2 pounds (2 x 3500 calories) should be lost by our lucky dieter in the first week alone.

We'll even set aside the truth that the quality of life of a person restricting themselves from food so severely is usually quite poor--they often feel listless, moody and depressed from deliberately starving themselves.

Okay, if the math provided by calorie-counting nutritionists is indeed correct, our dieter theoretically lost 2 pounds that first week. So far, so good...now let's continue onward. After a full year on the most popular restricted-calorie diet in the world today, here's what an average person's results *should* look like if limiting our caloric intake actually works...

1000 calorie deficit per day x 365 days in a year = 365,000 fewer calories not consumed over the course of the year.

365,000 calories divided by 3500 calories per pound of fat = **104 pounds**.

Therefore, the prey, errrr, client should have lost fully **104 lbs.** of body weight during that year of restricting calories.

Yet the average weight loss by *actual* human beings on this exact restricted-calorie diets is about *6-8 lbs.* after a full 12 MONTHS of daily, 1000-calorie per day deprivation!

And at the end of 24 months — two full years — the *predicted weight loss* on the highly popular 1000-calorie per day deficit should be a total of **208 lbs**!

Yet, the average *actual* total weight loss after two years on a restricted calorie diet is a ridiculous *4-5 lbs*!

In other words, they suffered horribly for twenty four months of their life and at the end of the second year they weigh, on average, a couple of pounds *more* than at the end of the first year on their restricted-calorie diet!

During year two, they ate another 365,000 FEWER calories than required for their normal energy needs — and the net result was that they GAINED weight!

And, of course, it's universally known that once they finally go off their Calorie-Restricted Diet not only will they immediately gain back the handful of pounds they managed to lose, they will soon weigh a good bit *more* than when they started down this miserable path.

"Eating less doesn't work. Weight loss achieved in trials of calorie-restricted diet is 'so small as to be clinically insignificant."
— Cochrane Collaboration, 2002

How Come Michael Phelps Doesn't Weigh 3523 Pounds?!

Let's consider the absurdity of the calories-in, calories-out fallacy from the exact opposite direction. You've surely heard of Olympic champion and world-record holder Michael Phelps.

And you may have heard that he famously puts away some 12,000 calories per day, a staggering number by any measure.

Now, the dude does exercise a lot — it's what he does for a living — but he only trains about 4 hours per day, not around the clock!

Elite swimmers don't even race at 100% of their max

all the time...the bulk of what they do in practice is grinding out mile after mile for hour after hour.

Even so, Michael Phelps burns upwards of 500 calories per hour, meaning that he expends about 2000 calories in his daily workout.

The rest of the day he spends doing as little as he can—resting and sleeping as much as possible so his body can recover.

So here's my question to all the calorie-counting nutrititionists out there: Where in the hell are the *extra 10,000 calories* per day going?!

Michael Phelps is ripped, so it's surely not going to store any fat on his 6'4", 195 lb. frame. Of course, Phelps isn't literally doing nothing the whole rest of the day—he's walking around, Tweeting, checking out the ladies, whatever it is he does—so let's (generously) give him credit for another 2000 calories just for being alive and listening to his iPod. That still leaves *8000 unaccounted for calories*. Per day!

According to the very math used to this very day by the very nutty Calorie-Counting Brigade, Michael Phelps is accumulating a caloric build-up of 8000 calories x 7 days = *56,000 extra calories* on a weekly basis.

Divided by their hallowed number of 3500 calories per pound, this should mean (again, according to *their* cartoon math, not according to anything resembling actual math or science) Michael Phelps is gaining 56,000 calories weekly divided by 3500 calories per pound = **16 pounds per week**.

In other words, if their little calorie theory is true, Michael Phelps *must gain 16 pounds* each and every week of the year.

That means that in the span between the 2008 and 2012 summer Olympic Games, Phelps *should* have gained 16 pounds x 208 total weeks = **3328 pounds!**

(And that's not even counting his starting weight of 195 lbs.)

So unless Michael Phelps steps up to the pool at the next Olympics weighing 3328 + his starting weight of 195 = **3523 pounds**, then the "nutritionists" have just been plain...ummm...*wrong* about this all along. Which is, of course, the case.

Calories-In does not *equal Calories-Out...or vice versa!* The sooner you let go of that notion, the sooner you can put yourself on track to make some real changes in your life and waistline.

If you want to discover the detailed science behind why the caloric theory of weight gain is rubbish and learn about the mountains of scientific evidence disproving it, I highly encourage you to pick up a copy of Gary Taubes' most excellent book, *Good Calories, Bad Calories*.

And if you still have even the slightest glimmer of belief in the Myth of the Reduced-Calorie Diet, I invite you to type the link below into your preferred Internet browser and watch a charming, hour-long presentation by anti-obesity crusader Zoë Harcombe.

Ms. Harcombe presents a devastating critique of reduced-calorie plans and cites nearly *100 scientific papers, studies and references* along the way to bolster her arguments...which are made all the more compelling by her fetching English accent!

http://www.zoeharcombe.com/2011/05/calories-energy-balance-thermodynamics-weight-loss/

"The much publicized diets with emphasis solely on calories are fallacious. It is excess carbohydrates and not calories only that

make a fat man fat."
—Dr. Richard Mackarness

Lie #2: We're Overweight Because We Don't Burn Enough Calories

The truth is: *Exercise alone doesn't make us lose weight.*

This second damned lie of weight loss seems to have been designed specifically as a CYA (Cover Yo' Ass) for government officials and the diet industry when we didn't actually lose any weight following their low-calorie regime.

Their argument basically goes like this: "Yeah, sure, you ate nothing but super low-calorie, low-fat foods and carbohydrates for the last five years in a row, but you didn't exercise enough and that's why you didn't lose any weight. It's not our fault...it's yours. Now join a gym and hit the treadmill!"

Shows like "Biggest Loser" reinforce this second damned lie of weight loss—that all we need to do is work out more and we'll shed pounds like a chicken shedding its feathers every fall.

I mean, sure, if we were able to live full-time in an artificial world like the "Biggest Loser" where the only thing we had to do each day was wake up and work out with the best personal trainers in the world and eat food cooked by professional chefs who carefully controlled every bite we ate, we would no doubt lose some weight.

But this pampered lifestyle isn't realistic, practical or sustainable for an average human being.

The "Biggest Loser" has become the poster child in the United States for the efficacy of the low-calorie/high work-out lifestyle that is supposed to lead us to the promised land of becoming magically fit and trim once again. However, it doesn't always work even

42

for them.

I won't name names, but if you were to look up some of the show's participants from previous seasons and find out where they are now, you would discover that a great number of them gained some of the weight back, and several of them—including even past winners of the show, who are supposedly the very best examples in the world of the success of the low-calorie fad—are right back where they started and weigh just as much or more than they ever did.

Don't get me wrong, I'm all for moving our bodies and shaking our booty on a regular basis, and I'm going to suggest that the more we play, the better we feel and the better we look. Not necessarily because of the calories we burn, but because simply getting off our butts helps reconnect us with our bodies.

Yet I also believe we can accomplish this without *all* the highly structured, artificial "exercise" and "work-out" baggage that supports the modern-day fitness center industry.

We'll revisit the topics of calories-in (low-calorie eating) and calories-out (high-quantity exercise) before long, but first let's touch on the third damned lie of weight loss.

Lie #3: We're Overweight Because We Eat Fat

The truth is: *Fat doesn't make us fat.*

In 2009 Robert Lustig, MD gave a powerful talk called *Sugar: The Bitter Truth*, in which he forcefully argued that our sugary diets are the cornerstone of the global obesity epidemic.

Dr. Lustig explained how the low-fat fad that's been actively promoted by the U.S. government and the media has succeeded in lowering our intake of fat from 40% to 30% of total calories.

Yet at the same time we've been eating less fat,

obesity levels have *grown* disproportionately during the years of the low-fat craze because most people substitute sugars or carbohydrates (which I often refer to as Mega-Sugars), for the fat they cut out of their diet.

Despite its name, fat itself doesn't make us fat any more than cold weather gives us colds or butterflies in our stomach are made of actual butterflies.

Fat contains calories. So does protein. Yet, as we will soon discover, neither fat nor protein have anything whatsoever scientifically to do with how our body stores and maintains fat.

Our bodies create fat out of excess glucose in our bloodstream. Only carbohydrates (whether as simple sugars or Mega-Sugars) create the excess glucose that gets stored inside our cells as fat.

Now let's take up the last of the damned lies that have been foisted upon us by the media and Big Diet...

Lie #4: We're Overweight Because We Have Faulty Genes

The truth is: *Our genes don't make us fat.*

This lie is arguably the worst one of all because it implies there's not a damn thing we can do about our weight other than blame our parents or curse biology.

I call it the Blame It On Mom excuse!

At least the low-calorie silliness gave us *something* to do—even if that something was the dopey recommendation to come as close as possible to starving ourselves to death!

The bad-genes fad suggests we have no hope at all and so we might as well give up and go out to dinner at the All-You-Can-Eat Carb Buffet every night of the week.

The good news is that—like every one of the other "Damned Lies of Weight Loss"—blaming our weight on our genes is both a damned and a passing fad.

Yet the myth of us being slaves to our own genes is so pervasive in the media, and this is such an important topic to grasp, that we should spend a few moments together exploring this topic before moving on.

By way of warning, we might get a little science-y here, but it's all for good cause, it's all for *you*! So stay with me—it'll be worth it!

We Are Communities of Cells

We are each of us merely communities of cells...some 65 or so trillion of them working together (some of the time!) to make up who we are.

Each and every one of our cells comes equipped with a nucleus that stores the cell's DNA.

The DNA is sort of like the cell's hard drive, containing a collection of programs that can be "run" when the cell receives a signal to do so...or not run if it never receives the signal.

But these initial programs are merely the *starting point* for what our cells can do and become. Despite what we've been led to believe, our cells are not "stuck" with only our initial programs for the rest of their existences. Indeed, our cells are quite brilliant at learning new skills and developing new "programs" for future behaviors.

You may have heard of this little thing called Evolution. Well, this is where *all* evolution happens—on a cellular level! When our cells learn, they evolve...and we evolve along with them. Our cells constantly monitor their micro-environment and adjust themselves accordingly—changing their own "programming" to adapt to changes that are happening around them.

If the environment around one of our cells becomes, say, too acidic, the cell will strive to find nearby alkaline sources in order to balance out its pH.

Even more incredibly, our cells don't just evolve, they pass on their learnings to their offspring, which in turn learn new stuff and evolve in new ways, and then pass on a different version of itself to its offspring and so on.

If some overly acidic cells in our thighs discover they can leech calcium phosphate from a nearby hip bone in order to correct their pH level, the cells that later come along to replace them will already know exactly how to do that same task as soon as they are "born".

In this fashion, little by little, our genetic code ebbs and flows over the years.

In fact, if we weren't able to learn and change at a cellular level in response to our local environment, none of us would be able to make it through a single day, much less a whole lifetime!

As Dr. Bruce Lipton writes in his classic book, *The Biology of Belief*, "The cell's operations are primarily molded by interaction with the environment, not by its genetic code."

Our Genes Learn, Change and Grow

When we provide a healthy environment for our cells, they thrive. When we provide a toxic environment for our cells, they get sick. The good news is that when we restore a healthy environment, our cells can and do recover and thrive once again.

Dr. Lipton notes, "Our genes are constantly being remodeled in response to life experiences. My research offers incontrovertible proof that biology's most cherished tenets regarding genetic determinism are fundamentally flawed."

Genetic determinism is just fancy scientist-talk for "my genes made me do it", and he argues persuasively in his work that this simply is *not true*.

While our genes *do* predispose us to certain physical characteristics and features, we all possess the ability to change and evolve right down to the cellular level.

The "Problem" With Identical Twins

Identical twins are sometimes held up as proof (especially by people who receive their medical training from glossy monthly magazines, lulz!) that we are merely products of our genes.

In fact, the real-world experiences of identical twins was one of the nails in the coffin of the old-fashioned theory that everything we do in our entire life is influenced directly by the genes we're born with.

As we've noted, the genes in everybody's cells learn and adapt and change, and this includes the subset of the population known as identical twins.

At birth, the DNA scans of identical twins are indeed identical. If you print a map of their genes onto clear plastic sheets and overlay them, they line up so exactly that they seem to be one and the same. There's nothing earth-shaking about that factoid, of course. The really interesting part comes later, after a lifetime of growth and adaptation on a cellular level. As life goes on for identical twins, their genes inevitably evolve separately and their DNA drifts further and further apart.

Spain has become an global leader in researching the genetic code of identical twins. In one typical example, a pair of identical twin sisters had settled down in the same small town in Spain.

Not only did they live in the same town, they lived just a couple of doors from each other on the very same street, and they shared, to all outward appearances, what seemed to be very similar lives.

So similar that Spanish scientists expected when the sister's genes were compared later in life they would remain nearly identical--maybe not an exact match, but very close to one.

Yet it turned out that even sharing almost identical lifestyles resulted in such completely different "choices" by each sister's genes that when they underwent a DNA scan in their sixties, the differences between the two sets of genes were so dramatic that researchers at first refused to believe they really were identical twins.

Only when the sisters were brought into the university laboratory and personally interviewed did the scientists on the project begrudgingly admit that despite their vast differences on the inside, the sisters still looked pretty darn identical on the outside.

"Genes are not destiny!" Bruce Lipton writes. "Environmental influences, including nutrition, stress and emotions, can modify those genes."

This means that none of us, not even identical twins, are slaves to our genes.

We will explore the concept of who we are on a cellular level and what it means to be a community of cells working together towards a common goal in much greater depth in Part Two of the *Low Carb Revolution.*

The primary takeaway for now is that regardless of what our mother or father, or even siblings, happen to look like, we *can* create our own unique physical expression of ourselves in the world.

In short, each of has the potential to be the Marilyn Munster of our own family!

Eminent cell biologist and medical researcher, Bruce Lipton, Ph.D., remarks how his fellow scientists and biologists have long been aware that we're *not* programmed by our genes as was once believed. Indeed, Dr. Lipton penned his ground-breaking book, *The Biology of Belief,* specifically for the rest of us.

Lipton writes: "99% of the rest of the population, the

'lay audience', is still operating from antiquated and disempowering beliefs about being victims of their genes."

How Are You Doing?

I want to thank you again for being here! Seriously, thank you! I love your willingness to stay with me and continue rediscovering yourself within these pages. Now you are about to gain an incredible appreciation for your body that has the potential to change the way you eat and how much you weigh forever!

By the time you finish reading the next few Keys, you will finally understand the exact mechanism of how we get fat and how we stay fat!

This is exciting stuff that can make an immediate and permanent impact on your life and your waistline. So let's roll up our sleeves and keep going, shall we?!

> *"The first thing to realize is that it is carbohydrate (starch and sugar) and carbohydrate only which fattens fat people."*
> —Richard Mackarness, MD

KEY #4:
"Appreciate Your Body Day"

It's Like Your Very Own Holiday!

I am about to ask you to do something unusual.

Mind you, this probably won't be the last time! Throughout this book I am going to ask you to *think* many unusual thoughts, to *feel* many unusual feelings, to *know* many unusual things and to take more than your fair share of unusual *actions*!

And by "unusual" I simply mean *different* from your previous experiences. Because it's about time you do things a little bit differently, wouldn't you agree?!

If you are currently carrying excess pounds in any part of your body, then what you've been doing up until now probably hasn't been a complete and total success...yet.

If you still haven't reached your birthright and natural state of your Ideal Body, then you still have more steps left on your journey...and the steps still ahead of you are no doubt the most important ones of all.

Some of these steps we'll take together in the *Low Carb Revolution* are about the things we put into our bodies — the foods we eat and the foods we don't eat. But other steps will involve how we feel, what we say to ourselves, what we think about ourselves, and, ultimately, how we treat ourselves.

So let's kick off the unusualness right now with your very own holiday. I call it...

Appreciate Your Body Day

Holidays come and holidays go, but I really cannot think of a better reason to celebrate than to show appreciation for our wonderful bodies--these magnificent creations that endure so much use and abuse and yet somehow manage to keep on trucking day after day.

Our journey towards our Ideal Body (whatever that means to you...whether a number, a shape or a good feeling about yourself!) requires that we reconnect Body with Mind, that we take the time out of our busy schedules to put the two of them in the same room together so they can begin communicating again, and rebuild what has in all likelihood become a dysfunctional relationship.

The work you and I are doing together here is basically Couples Counseling for our Mind and Body!

As part of the Appreciate Your Body Day festivities, we're going to create two very special celebrations. These celebrations are opportunities for our Mind and Body to come together and play games and reconnect with one another. (I often use the word "game" here and elsewhere because Mind loves playing games *and* Body loves playing games.)

But make no mistake, this is the Work. These games are the Work.

You want to lose your excess weight? You want to heal? You want to wake up and finally get here? You want to let your light shine in the world like never before?

Then play these games. Then do this work.

By the way, we'll be doing a lot more profound self-exploration and healing together in Part Two of the *Low*

Carb Revolution, this is just a taste of things to come!

> *"Without deviations from the*
> *norm, progress is not possible."*
> —Frank Zappa

Celebration 1: The Body Bath

To kick off the Appreciate Your Body Day festivities, we're going to take a bath.

Not just any bath, mind you. Today—hopefully you'll make *today* the day for your very own holiday…I mean, why put off celebrating yourself until tomorrow or next week or the next lifetime?!—we're going to take a super-special Body Bath.

To start, prepare your bath as usual. Add bubbles or don't add bubbles, whatever you like. Next, get naked. This is something we all do too little of—just being with our bodies, on our own, without any clothes to hide behind. (Mark Sisson, a leading light in the Paleo movement, has a wonderful, informal definition for his Ideal Body: "To look good naked!")

Now ease into the bath. Then hold up, for example, your right hand. And *say* to your right hand words to the effect of: "Right hand, I just wanna say thank you. I appreciate you and I love you so much. You've picked up so many things for me in my life…and you've dropped other things I didn't want to hold on to…and you wrote down all those lovely words for me…and you throw balls really well…and I would like to tell you thank you, thank you, thank you!"

Say all this out loud, so your right hand can revel in the fact that it's being singled out for praise and thanks in front of your whole body.

And then move on to the next body part—your knees, your breasts, your toes. Your fingernails, your bum, your earlobes and your tongue. Omit nothing. Praise everything.

The entire point here is to celebrate and love your beautiful body *exactly the way it is right now...not as it may one day become.*

After all, if you had a little daughter, you wouldn't say to her, "Oh, honey, I can't wait for you to grow up and become an astronaut—I'm gonna love you so much when you go into space!" No! You tell her that you love her right now, just the way she is. What she becomes later has no bearing on your love for her now!

And it's no different with your body. The journey to returning to your Ideal Body starts with loving your body exactly as it is right now. And when you're in love with somebody, you tell them, right?!

So we're gonna tell our body we love it—every gorgeous, sexy, perfect bit of it. And not just on the outside, but the inside as well.

Shower your heart with love, your kidneys with thanks, your stomach with forgiveness and your small intestine with gratitude.

Out loud, praise your pancreas for secreting the hard-working hormones that keep you alive.

Admire your Insulin for helping you store fat in your body. Give love and thanks and encouragement to your fat-burning hormone Glucagon and your appetite-suppressing hormone of Leptin.

Remember to thank your bones—even the old, creaky, stiff ones...hell, *especially* thank the afflicted ones because they have such a tough job to do and they still keep doing it day upon day to the best of their ability.

Take your time with your Body Bath. Linger over your body and connect with it intimately.

Modern humans spend so little time in the space I refer to as "Non-sexual nudity," just admiring and appreciating our bodies the way they are right now.

For most of us, the only time we ever get naked for prolonged periods of time is when we're expressing our sexuality.

And, as often as not, that means a darkened room and hiding under the covers and lots of self-judgments and negative inner-dialogue about what our lover must be thinking about our bodies.

Yet how can we expect others to love our bodies until we discover how to love them ourselves?! So that's the Body Bath.

Do this today, if at all possible. Believe me, your body *longs* to hear you say nice things about it and thank it for all its hard work!

Celebration 2: The Altar of You

The festivities of Appreciate Your Body day continue with our second celebration: the creation of an Altar to *You*.

Start by marking off a space to put your altar. You don't need to rush out to Altars-R-Us and buy a pre-made piece of furniture or anything.

Simply draping a scarf over the top of a waist-high bookcase or something similar is plenty fine. Once you've created an altar space, we're going to put a few items on it.

A **candle**. Every altar needs a candle, right?!

A **heart**. This can be a little plastic heart from the local dollar store or a heart-shaped rock or a heart charm from a charm bracelet. Even drawing a simple heart shape on an index card works fine.

A **mirror**. After all, this is an Altar to You, so we want to include *you* in the experience!

Something from **nature**. This could be a rock or a shell or that two-toned feather you picked up the other day. (It's very common for people to already have some things from nature they'd previously found at the beach or in the woods and just didn't quite know what it was for until they set up their personal altar!)

A representation of an **animal**. This could be in the form of a little plastic figure of an animal or a clay statue or anything at all. It can represent a real animal from nature, like Bear or Monkey, or it can be an "imaginary" animal like Dragon or Unicorn. This animal represents your Spirit Animal, which is always with you to help protect and support you during the struggles and the successes of your life.

These are all the initial objects you need to include in your Altar to You, but of course feel free to add any other items that you feel belong there.

If you feel strongly about a particular religious faith, you may also want to place a representation of your faith on the altar—a cross, a statue of the Buddha, etc.

Now that our personal altar is set up, here's how to use it...whenever you have a question or need help making a decision, approach your altar.

Stand before the altar and say something to the effect of, "I'm trying to decide between X and Y. If I loved myself the most, which would I decide?" Then stop and listen for a response.

Say you're trying to decide whether your body would prefer taking a yoga class or going to Zumba. Discover the answer by asking your body directly in front of the Altar of You.

When you're trying to establish what number or dress size or image of yourself will represent your Ideal Body, go consult the Altar of You. When you've lost a few crucial pounds, go to the Altar of You and just let out a big sigh of thanks! And especially make time to visit the Altar of You in order to forgive yourself...and love yourself...and praise yourself for having the courage to continue exploring the road less traveled!

Remembering to Love Yourself

Taking a Body Bath isn't something we just do once. We can repeat this loving, self-affirming experience as often as we desire.

Similarly, we should add new items to our personal Altar and consult our own highest wisdom on a regular basis. Let's never lose of the most important "science" of all: *The more we love ourselves the more things fall into place in every aspect of our lives.*

That means loving our minds and goals and dreams. And it means loving the physical packaging it all comes in — our spectacular, unique, wonderful bodies.

A part of you may find this whole concept of celebrating an Appreciate Your Body day to be the height of silliness.

But, trust me, your *body* won't. Your body will love every second of this experience.

And since our body is where most of us actually *keep* our excess weight, it's probably a good idea to start developing a more fun, loving and even silly relationship with our body, wouldn't you agree?!

Hey, maybe we'll even have an Appreciate Your Mind day later on. But for now this is all about your body — so don't let your mind talk you out of playing this important game!

> *"You are NOT what you eat,*
> *you are WHAT YOU DO with*
> *what you eat."*
> — Robert Lustig, MD

KEY #5:
"The Language of Your Body"

Your Body Doesn't Speak Words

You and I communicate to other people and even to ourselves largely through words and language.

But when your body goes to talk to itself, it doesn't, of course, speak English or Chinese or any other human languages. Instead it uses electrical impulses and neuro-transmitters for seriously urgent messages that need to arrive within milliseconds or less—like sending a signal to jerk your fingers backwards if they accidentally stray into the flame of a candle.

In addition, your body deploys chemical messengers called hormones that travel at a much more leisurely pace and which can carry a great deal more information than electrical signals.

The messages within your body that concern themselves with the making and the storing of fat are sent via hormones, and so that's the language we're going to turn our attention to here.

We won't be learning the entire language of chemical messages called hormones—not by a long shot. We're just gonna learn enough to get by!

You know how before you travel to France or Italy you brush up on a couple of French or Italian phrases that you'll be needing to say when you get there?!

So that's what we're going to do—we're going to learn a few important phrases of Hormone-Speak so we can *tell* our own body some really cool things we'd like it to do, or not do, from now on.

Because wouldn't it be delightful if we could speak the body's exact language and tell it, "Oh, no, monsieur, pleez do not make any fat from ze food I am eating!"

Communication is Everything

For realz, communication is the name of the game! Most of our problems stem directly from the fact that we don't know how to communicate with either our bodies *or* our minds!

Throughout the *Low Carb Revolution* we're going to discover ways to communicate with our bodies and with our minds better than ever before in our lives.

And—and this is a huge "and"—we're going to discover how to put our minds and our bodies in communication with one another. And that is gonna change the game entirely, my friends!

Now I'd love to be able to tell you that your body speaks Post-It™ notes, and that if you leave enough of them on your bathroom mirror or refrigerator with messages about losing excess weight that your body will eventually get the message.

But it doesn't work that way, alas. Post-It™ notes are written by our minds and read by our minds, but not by our bodies.

A while back a private client came to me for a smoking-cessation session. After we did our magic together, she remarked, "I'm also thinking about losing weight." I replied, "That's great. But the problem is, the weight's not in your thoughts and *thinking* about losing weight is of no particular value one way or the other."

Bottom line: If it were possible to simply "Think Ourselves Thin" with the brain in our heads, every last one of us would've already done so long ago.

I mean, duh!

That said, our minds *are* capable of many wondrous things — even more than you might now realize, as we'll discover in Part Two.

But first things first, let's start by laying the foundation for learning how the body speaks to itself.

The Language of Hormones

There are hundreds, if not thousands, of separate systems operating within our extraordinarily complicated bodies 24 hours a day that require constant monitoring and tweaking.

Our pH balance, our blood sugar, our oxygen levels, our core temperature, on and on. Many of these systems flourish only within exceedingly narrow parameters with very little margin for error.

You've no doubt heard of hormones, if only because of how much they are said to "run amuck" during our teenage years. Hormones are chemical messengers that deliver information from one part of our body to another.

These chemical communications are generally created by a gland in one area of the body and then sent to deliver their message in a completely different area.

Here's what is important to know about hormones: most hormones have only a limited number of possible messages (sometimes only one) that they deliver to a limited number of other organs or systems (again, sometimes only one.)

Let's use a metaphor to understand how the "language of hormones" works within us...

As you may recall from history class or watching *Bill & Ted's Excellent Adventure*, Troubadours were traveling musicians in the Middle Ages who wandered around playing songs about love and chivalry and all that jazz.

Actually, playing music was more of a hobby for

them—the real job of Troubadours wasn't quite so glamorous.

Long before the Internet, network news, mobile phones, newspapers or even CB radios, news was spread from one region of the kingdom to another via the Troubadours.

Whenever a Troubadour showed up in a village, everybody gathered 'round to discover the news of the day—and by news of the day I mean the news of however many months or even years it had been since the last Troubadour had passed through.

Thus at the feet of the medieval Troubadours did the townspeople learn of the death of kings, the birth of princes, the triumphs or tragedies of war, the recent laws that had been enacted and all the latest scandals of those scoundrels at the high court.

One Troubadour, One Message

Now for the sake of understanding how our body communicates with itself, let's pretend that instead of recounting *all* the general news of the land, the Troubadours of old had a rule where they could only deliver one type of news.

For example, let's say you were a medieval Troubadour (and who's to say you weren't?!) and your only job was to announce to the populace when the King had died.

Obviously, until the King actually died you would have very little to do other than sit around and think up new songs to sing while you were a-journeying, and maybe play the recently invented game of chess with your fellow Troubadours.

Now, let's say the King finally dies...and good riddance, we never liked the old bastard anyway!

So you hurry out into the kingdom and give everyone the happy news and there's a party in every village and your new songs are quite the hit.

Exhausted, you return home and prepare to be sent out again. In due course, the King's sons betray and poison one another and his eldest daughter unexpectedly becomes Queen. So you don your jerkin (what we nowadays would call a "vest") to go tell everybody the news, but alas, it turns out a completely different Troubadour is tasked with the job of traveling about the kingdom to let everybody know a new monarch has ascended to the throne.

And that's *their* only job...the only message this other Troubadour ever gets to share is to tell people when a new King or Queen has been anointed — or be-sainted, or whatever the hell it is they do with Kings or Queens to make it official!

And you only get to venture out and share the news when the monarch has died, so you patiently wait for the Queen to kick the bucket.

When the Queen raises taxes the following year, it's your friend Reginald who gets to go tell the rest of the kingdom. When she grants a tax-free year following that, it's your arch-enemy Stephanus who delivers that news. And so on.

In other words, each Troubadour has one primary message to communicate.

The result is that over time when the villagers see you coming, they already know the news. You're the one who always comes with the message: "The King is dead, long live the King."

You don't even have to say anything to the villagers — just a glimpse of you is all they need to know the news.

In other words, the Troubadour himself *is* the message.

Now this isn't a particularly efficient system, but it is a capital idea when you don't have the luxury of words or language, which, again, is the case with our bodies.

Our Inner Troubadours

Our hormones act very much like medieval Troubadours with only a single message to deliver. We have lots and lots of these Inner Troubadours to carry different messages to all the many unfathomably complex systems in our bodies.

Generally, one Troubadour (hormone) goes out to inform a specific system or gland that it should begin doing a particular action.

Later, a completely *different* Troubadour (that is to say, a separate hormone) shows up to announce when the system or gland should *stop* doing whatever it's been doing.

Since our primary concern here is discovering how our body tells itself to store fat and how it tells itself to release fat, the first two "phrases" we're going to learn in Hormone-Speak Lexicon will cover exactly that!

By now you have surely divined that we must also have two separate Troubadours within us who are each charged with spreading a single message about what to do with the fat in our bodies.

One Troubadour carries the message: "Store fat! Store fat!"

The second Troubadour has the opposite message: "Burn fat! Burn fat!"

The "formal" names of these two Troubadours who each carry a single, vitally important message are Insulin and Glucagon...which sound rather like character names from a play by Shakespeare! (*"Alas, fair Glucagon, yon lies poor Insulin, witlessly hoisted by his own petard."*)

Without further ado, let's meet hapless Insulin and feckless Glucagon up close and personal!

*"All truths are easy to
understand once they're
discovered; the point is to
discover them."*
—Galileo

KEY #6:
"How We Got Fat"

A Tale of Two Troubadours

My brothers and sisters, we have arrived at a moment of truth. In this Key and the next, we will discover not only the secret of how we get fat, but also the two vitally important phrases in Hormone-Speak we can use to either start or stop that process.

The crazy thing is that these easy-to-learn phrases are *still* a big secret to so many people.

We've already found out that this so-called "secret" was originally discovered over 150 years back by Mr. William Banting, and the science behind that secret was largely determined by his descendent Dr. Frederick Banting going on 90 years ago!

So we have a pair of Troubadours — which, again, is just my poetic name for the chemical messengers that fancy scientists with their fancy Ph.D.'s and their mismatched argyle socks call hormones — within us, and these Troubadours are entirely responsible for the fat we gain and the fat we lose in our cells.

Without further ado…[Insert blare of trumpets here, lol!]… let's meet them now!

I give to you…Insulin and Glucagon, They are our Inner Troubadours who are respectively sent out to inform our cells to either add fat or let go of fat.

When they're not circulating through our blood system, our Troubadours hang out in their Shakespearean-sounding (again!) homeland called the *islets of Langerhans*, which is located in the kingdom of Pancreas. (Have I mentioned lately that you can't make this stuff up?!)

However Insulin and Glucagon are rarely idle. As we'll discover in Key #7, one or the other of these Troubadours is almost *continuously* being dispatched into our bloodstream depending on the level of our blood sugar...which itself is constantly and obsessively monitored, tweaked and re-tested by our bodies. Insulin and Glucagon are responsible for delivering just a single message—each of which goes to the heart of the process of gaining or losing weight.*

(The actual biochemical mechanism of gaining/losing fat involves complex interactions between fatty acids, lipids, protein cascades, triglycerides and other complex stuff I'm not gonna burden you with because it doesn't really add anything to our conversation about losing weight...in the same way that you don't need to know the physics behind how lasers work in order to use a DVD player; you simply need to know how to push Play, Pause, Rewind, etc.)

Say Hello to Insulin!

Insulin was a rather lonely little Troubadour for the first 2 million years of human evolution.

Even though small amounts of Insulin are released whenever we eat *anything*, Insulin largely concerns itself with eliminating excess sugars from the bloodstream and storing them as fat—and up until very, very, very recently humans simply didn't consume enough sugars for Insulin to have much to do on a regular basis.

As recently as 1900, Americans consumed an average of about **one pound** of added sugar in an entire year.

The hormone Insulin had an easy job of it back then, venturing out only now and again to scoop up any extra sugar—which is called glucose once it's broken down in our bloodstream.

Since our fair Troubadour's mission is to keep the glucose OUT of our blood, not only does Insulin store the glucose in our cells as fat, it also stands guard over that stored fat in order to prevent it from escaping back into the bloodstream again.

In this fashion, the added sugars in our blood are eliminated and the narrow range of our internal blood sugar is neatly maintained.

"Some of the glucose is converted to glycogen to be used for immediate energy needs. The body's ability to store or hold glycogen is limited to only a few hundred grams. The glucose that is not readily used or converted to glycogen is converted to fat."
—Morrison Bethea, MD, Sam Andrews, MD, Leighton Steward & Luis Balart, MD in *SUGAR BUSTERS!*

Now the more sugars we consume, the more glucose appears in our blood supply.

The more glucose that appears, the more Insulin is released to collar that nasty glucose, lock it up in our cells as triglycerides (fatty acids) and then *guard* it until such time as a famine comes along and that energy can be released and put to use.

Lehninger's *Principles of Biochemistry* is often referred to as the "Bible of Biochemistry".

If you go to the index and search for "How do we accumulate fat?", here is the answer you'll receive: "High blood glucose elicits the release of Insulin, which speeds the uptake of glucose by the tissues and favors the storage of fuels as glycogen and triacylglycerols, while inhibiting fatty acid mobilization in adipose tissue."

Translation: High glucose (which comes entirely from sugars and carbohydrates) calls Insulin into our bloodstream to store the excess glucose as glycogen (easily available energy in our livers) or triglycerides (difficult-to-access fatty acids) in our fat cells and then keeps it from escaping (mobilizing).

The problem is, for most Americans, those times of *famine* when we can burn off stored fat have become few and far between.

As in, never!

A Spoonful of Sugar

A pound of excess sugar per year for each American at the turn of the previous century became **five pounds** of added sugar each year by the end of World War II.

But even that amount was still pretty manageable for our tenacious Troubadour called Insulin, with his one "song" about ridding of glucose from the bloodstream.

Through World War II and even into 1970s and 1980s, the average American was not overweight and outright obesity was a rarity. Indeed, if you've tried my experiment of going back to watch feature films, TV shows and music videos from that era you'll be literally dumbstruck by how damn thin just about everybody seemed to be!

But a funny thing happened on the way to end of the decade.

> *"The excessive consumption of any sugars leads to health problems."*
> —Robert Lustig, MD

Sugar Nation

As the '80s drew to a close and the Fat Food industry exploded and High Fructose Corn Syrup (HFCS) became ubiqitious, Americans were by now consuming a stunning **75 pounds** of additional sugars per year! (That is to say, these were sugars in *addition* to any naturally occurring sugars in fruits, vegetables and the like!)

Our little Troubadour called Insulin now had his job cut out for him. He was constantly being summoned to snatch up as much glucose as possible from the blood and store it as fat in every nook and cranny it could find.

For 2 million years of human evolution, the last 200,000 of which were focused solely on perfecting the species called Homo Sapiens,

Insulin was the quiet, nerdy wallflower in the daily dance of life. For all that time Insulin mostly just stood around and watched all the other kids dancing.

Now, as the '80s wound down and Big Food pumped High Fructose Corn Satan into everything they could find and Chicken McNuggets were introduced on a nationwide basis and everything became available in a super-sized version, Insulin suddenly became the Belle of the Ball!

And Americans started becoming fatter. Like a lot fatter. Like really quickly.

But that was then and this is now. By 2010, the average American consumed a staggering **160 pounds of added sugar** per year.

That's an amount almost equal to the entire body weight of 165 pounds of the average American woman today! (Just by way of contrast, the average weight of an American woman as recently as WWII was closer to 130 pounds.)

No matter how you stack it, 160 pounds is a lot of sugar!

Picture, if you will, a 5 lb. bag of sugar, fairly bursting at the seams with crystalline, sugary goodness. Now imagine a pile of 32 of these 5 lb. bags of sugar — 160 pounds, all told — and you'll have a memorable picture of our average annual consumption of excess sugars in the United States today.

And with that kind of workload, the poor Troubadour responsible for grabbing up all that sugar and finding cells in which to stash it away as fat has become so overworked and so exhausted that we now face an epidemic of Type II Diabetes unprecedented in the history of the world.

Type II Diabetics have to regularly inject *extra Insulin* because their shell-shocked Inner Troubadour is basically just worn out and too exhausted to keep playing anymore.

So let's recap what we know about Insulin…

1) Insulin's primary job is to get rid of excess glucose from our bloodstream;

2) Insulin does this by storing the glucose as fat (in the form of triglycerides, or fatty acids) in cells throughout our body;

3) Since the job of Insulin is to keep the glucose *out* of our bloodstream completely, it doesn't just imprison the glucose in our cells, it also stands guard over the newly deposited fat in order to keep it from escaping.

4) The ONLY way for the fat to "escape" from its cell is to leave the way it came in — in other words, it must be converted from trigycerides back into glucose and only then can it return to the bloodstream and be "burned up" as energy. But, again, the ongoing *presence* of Insulin is like an ever-vigilant prison guard whose job is to prevent the prisoners (i.e., fatty acids) from ever escaping.

So the first "word" we've learned in Hormone-Speak is **Insulin**. And here's how our body interprets that word...

Insulin means, "Capture excess glucose in our bloodstream and imprison it in literal and figurative cells within our body...and then guard this stored fat with its life so the fat can't escape!"

Okay, that's the message Insulin carries. So far, so good!

Introducing Glucagon

Enter Glucagon, the unsung hero of our body. For the first 1,999,960 (out of 2,000,000!) years of human evolution, Glucagon was pretty much the most popular kid in school.

Like most of our Inner Troubadours, Glucagon also has one job and one job only.*

(Not to put too fine a point on it, but, again, I'm totally simplifying all of this for the specific conversation we're having about losing weight. Yes, Insulin and Glucagon also do other odd jobs for our body...and if microbiology is your passion, I strongly encourage you to explore the extracurricular hobbies and interests of these important hormones further!)

The one and only job that Glucagon performs is to go around and *liberate* the stored fats from their cells and set them free—back into our bloodstream, where they can be burned for energy.

Thus is Glucagon our swashbuckling Troubadour, liberating our fatty acids from their cellular imprisonment and allowing them the opportunity to finally escape from our bodies.

Glucagon's job is a heroic one. Once it makes sure the coast is clear, and that meddlesome bore Insulin is nowhere to be found, Glucagon throws open the prison doors of our cells and says, "Fly little fat deposits, fly away and be gone from here forever!"

So our second "word" in Hormone-Speak is **Glucagon**. *Glucagon means*, "Run around and liberate as much fat imprisoned in our cells as possible in order to burn it up as energy!"

> *"Living a healthy lifestyle will*
> *only deprive you of poor health,*
> *lethargy and fat."*
> —Jill Johnson

Hmmmm, Whom To Invite to the Dance?!

Knowing what you now know, whom—hey, how often do we get a chance to use "whom" in a sentence these days, lulz?!—do you think we should invite to the Dance in our body on a more frequent basis?!

Which of these two Inner Troubadours would best support our goal of losing weight?

Again, let's consider each in turn, starting with our old pal Insulin.

The primary message this overworked Troubadour delivers for us is to cause liver, muscle and fat tissue to store the glucose in our blood as fat.

After which Insulin actively stands guard over these stored fatty acids to prevent them from being released back into the blood supply and overwhelming us with too much glucose.

Of course, hoity-toity scientists with their fast cars and their blonde trophy wives don't use phrases like "stands guard over these stored fatty acids". Instead they use their own brainy-talk term of *lipolysis* and suchlike to describe Insulin's role in blocking the conversion of fat back into glucose.

By the way...we possess two main types of cells that

71

are capable of storing fat for us—our muscle cells (mycocytes) and our fat cells (adipocytes).

Together they account for about two-thirds of all the cells in our body.

Which leaves about one-third of us that doesn't have the ability to store any fat whatsover. This explains why our eyeballs, fingernails, brains and similar bits don't also get fatter along with the rest of us.

Meanwhile, when Glucagon gets a rare opportunity to venture out into our bloodstream to deliver its message, this dashing hormone assists in jail-breaking our stored fat back into the blood supply so it can be used for our immediate energy needs.

So Insulin stores the sugars and Mega-Sugars in our blood as fat and keeps it there, while Glucagon liberates the imprisoned fat and turns it back into glucose so we can get burn it as energy.

Have you made your decision about which of these Troubadours you'd like to spend more time with?

Fat-storing Insulin?

or

Fat-liberating Glucagon?

Keep in mind that these hormones are at exact odds with one another. You can only pick one to go to the dance with, not both. Have you made your decision?

If you chose to invite fat-liberating Glucagon to the Prom, then congratulations! You are well on your way to finally understanding how to let go of the fat in your body forever.

On the other hand, if you chose to invite fat-storing Insulin to the Prom instead, I strongly suggest you skip ahead to Part Two of the *Low Carb Revolution* and jump directly into the process of rebuilding your relationship with your beautiful body…and only once that process of transformation and healing is more advanced should you return to this section. Then we'll continue our journey of discovery together!

Okay, time to find out precisely *how* to invite our well-rested Glucagon to the dance of life anytime we desire.

To accomplish that, we're going to ask what I refer to as the $50 Billion Question! And we'll do this in the very next Key!

> *"Excess Insulin is killing people prematurely, and even those who survive to an older age often have a greatly reduced quality of life. The importance of Insulin has been ignored in the vast majority of nutritional and dietetic literature. The 'Insulin connection' needs to be understood and must be told over and over until it is appreciated."*
> —Leighton Steward, Sam Andrews, MD,
> Morrison Bethea, MD and Luis Balart, MD in
> *SUGAR BUSTERS!*

KEY #7:
"The $50 Billion Question"

Big Food and Big Diet Are In Bed Together

Of all the secrets, strategies and learnings you'll encounter in the *Low Carb Revolution*, this particular chapter is the one that Big Diet most fervently hopes you will skip.

Because it has the potential to put them out of business. A $50 billion a year business.

Let's be clear about this: Big Diet's business model does *not* entail helping anybody lose weight.

There's no money in people losing weight, because once they've lost it they have an annoying habit of no longer handing over their hard-earned money to Big Diet!

No, the money for Big Diet is in creating l*ifelong customers* who will pay handsomely, month after month, for the rest of their lives.

The money for Big Diet comes from creating product lines of "diet" foods that directly contribute to fat gain and storage in the purposefully misinformed people who purchase them.

Would you like to know another little secret that's been deliberately kept from us?

Big Food and Big Diet are just different divisions of the very same Multi-National Corporations.

The goal of the Big Food division in the corporation is to sell cheap, processed food that (quite conveniently) causes its customers to become fat. The goal of the Big Diet division in the exact same corporation is to market expensive, processed "diet" food to the fat customers created by its "rival" division.

I know this probably sounds a bit far-fetched and Kevin Trudeau-y, so let me share with you a few typical examples.

For instance, you may think of **Jenny Craig** as simply a weight-loss company. But to the shareholders of Société des Produits Nestlé S.A., *the largest food conglomerate in the world,* Jenny Craig is just another division in the company — the one responsible for the highly profitable Jenny's Cuisine "diet" product line, with more than *80 menu items* and growing.

Meanwhile, a competing division within the *very same* Nestlé Corporation is diet mammoth **Optifast**, which develops and markets extensive "diet" products of its own.

But wait, there's more! One of the pillars of Big Food in the United States is Kraft Foods, Inc., makers of the **South Beach** "diet" product line.

Weight Watchers is owned by a giant European consortium that owns or partially owns numerous Big Food multi-national corporations. And Weight Watchers reduced-calorie "diet" products are *exclusively* produced and distributed by the HJ Heinz Co., the $10 billion a year food giant.

Harold Katz, the founder of weight-loss behemoth **Nutrisystem**, made so much money by the mid-'80s that he retired from the diet business and bought a private jet along with the Philadelphia 76ers NBA franchise!

And guess who owns the ostensibly "low-carb" **Atkins** diet company? Atlanta-based Roark Capital Group, who also happen to be the proud owners of carbohydrate-heavy quick service chains like Cinnabon and Carvel!

Finally, Big Diet heavyweights such as **Nutrisystem** (Nasdaq: NTRI), **Medifast** (NYSE: MED) and **Herbalife** (NYSE: HLF) are all major corporations with a global reach and are publicly traded on the Nasdaq or New York Stock Exchange.

Increasingly, Big Food and Big Diet are ONE! With that understanding behind us, now let's ask ourselves the $50 Billion Question, the one these corporate fatcats do not want you to know the answer to.

How Can We Invite Glucagon to the Dance?

Recall our previous discovery that the *exclusive franchise* on storing fat in our cells is held by the hormone Insulin, and the *sole rights* of liberating that stored fat are owned by the hormone Glucagon.

So we want to determine how to extend an invitation to the ongoing dance in our body to fat-liberating Glucagon.

Because if we can figure this out, we'll no longer need Big Food/Diet and their $50 billion in yearly sales of "low-calorie, reduced-fat" products that are, frankly, very much part of the problem and not at all part of the solution.

In the previous chapter we learned that fat-storing Insulin is "called" when we have too much sugar in our blood.

The call goes something like this: "Yo, Insulin, wazzup?! We got all this extra glucose hanging around, dawg—we need you to come lock that shit up tight in our fat cells 'cause we can't burn it fast enough!"

Contrariwise, Glucagon's telephone only starts ringing when we have too *little* available glucose in our blood.

And that call might sound like this: "Get up off your lazy butt, Glucagon, and get down here fast! We need some energy and we need it now—so you gotta come bust out some of that nasty-ass fat that got stored away so we can finally put it to use for some damn energy!"

(Why exactly our body systems talk to one another like cartoon hoodlums is a modern medical mystery!)

As we've discussed previously, our body maintains many of our internal systems within a very precise range—and straying too far on either side of a baseline can lead to inconvenient outcomes like, oh, death. Systems such as our pH balance, core temperature, oxygen levels and, naturally, blood sugar, just to mention a few, are closely and constantly monitored by our bodies.

When our blood sugars grow too high, Insulin is "called" in to store the glucose as fatty acids in our cells and then stand vigilant guard over the fat so it won't escape.

When our blood sugar falls too low, Glucagon is "called" in to liberate the stored fat and turn it back into glucose so we can burn it up as energy.

And when our blood sugar is normal, a delicate ballet between Glucagon and Insulin ensues, a *pas de deux* of storing fat and burning fat according to our immediate energy needs.

For the first 1,999,960-odd years of human evolution, most people's blood sugar was normal most of the time.

We only started becoming obese when we had nonstop access to surplus sugars for our Insulin to convert into fat.

So the key to inviting Glucagon to spend more time in our bloodstream doing its lovely, lovely job of burning off our fat supplies is to maintain a normal blood sugar level.

> *"It is a hard matter, my fellow*
> *citizens, to argue with the belly,*
> *since it has no ears."*
> --Plutarch

The "Secret" to Losing Weight

Although this whole concept is somehow still a *secret* to most people, it's a secret that's been laying around in plain sight for so long that it's almost painful to contemplate how we could fail to notice and take action on it.

After all, we are in the midst of a literal, worldwide epidemic of obesity, Type II diabetes and other weight-related health problems.

But to this day we are told by "nutritionists" that the best (indeed, only) way to lose weight is to reduce the number of calories we consume.

They've repeated their demonstrably false Caloric Myth of Weight Loss so often that they sometimes refer to it as nutritional *science*...which is an oxymoron of the highest order! According to the *actual* science of biology, here's what *really* takes place within our bodies every single day of our lives:

When our blood sugar is high, Insulin is called. Insulin stores the excess blood sugar as fat and guards it so that it can't escape.

When our blood sugar is low, Glucagon is called. Glucagon sets free the glucose stored as fat so it can be immediately burned up by the body as energy.

To recap what actual science tells us about the mechanism for gaining weight...

High blood sugar -> Insulin -> weight gain
Low blood sugar -> Glucagon -> weight loss

Notice that there's *nothing* whatsoever in the

formula about calories! Neither Insulin nor Glucagon care about calories—they can't even *spell* calories!

All that either hormone cares about is the *level of our current blood sugar.*

If we eat or drink something with little or no sugars, the calories in it are prioritized and processed almost immediately as energy. Almost no Insulin is called and no fat is created in the absence of sugars (or so-called Mega-Sugars) in the food or drink we consume. The *only* way to create and store fat in our bodies is with the hormone Insulin.

The *only* way to liberate and release stored fat in our bodies is with the hormone Glucagon.

Yes, Virginia, it *is* that simple!

Fat storage and fat release are not "regulated" by calories any more than calories cause us to grow hair (that's done by the hormone Testosterone) or calories cause us to grow taller (all the credit here goes to Growth Hormone) or calories make us lactate after having a baby (thank you, Oxytocin).

The level of our blood sugar alone determines whether Insulin is called or Glucagon is called. Our blood sugar is *not* influenced by the amount of "calories" we eat, but only by the amount of sugars contained in the food and drink we introduce into our bodies.

If the amount of sugars we consume are low, we lose weight…if the amount of sugars we consume are high, we gain.

There is no other mechanism in our physical body for storing fat or for losing fat than this.

The Holy Grail

So we're almost there! We've almost reached the promised land. Just one final big chunk to understand and all the pieces of the weight-loss puzzle will finally fall into place.

When this happens it will be a moment in your life when you finally *get* it! Everything about the times in the past when you tried and tried to lose weight and failed spectacularly will suddenly make sense.

The times in your life when you ate less food than would sustain a freakin' pygmy mouse and you still gained weight will make sense. The times in your life when you went out of your way to overeat and you somehow didn't gain a single extra pound will also make sense. It's just all gonna make such sense to you!

And there's a question I sincerely hope you are asking yourself right about now. It's a question that, once answered, has the potential to take you from where you are now in your weight-loss journey back to your birthright and your natural state of living and thriving in your Ideal Body. That question is...

"Is there anything I can personally do to 'call' the hormone Glucagon into bloodstream so I can get rid of my existing fat while avoiding calling the hormone Insulin which stores and guards body fat?!"

To which I shall respond...

"Excellent question, thanks for asking. And, as a matter of fact, there *is* something you can do on a regular basis to invite Glucagon rather than Insulin to the daily dance of being you!"

And that's exactly what we're going to learn next!

"Unhealthy living is the reason
why you feel burned out,
fatigued, prematurely old and
full of aches and pains."
—Paul C. Bragg

KEY #8:
"The Glycemic Index"

"You Talking to Me?!"

Later in the book we'll explore our almost incessant habit of talking to ourselves all day long.

Of course, talking to ourselves isn't the real problem. The problem is the typically negative, self-defeating and downright mean-spirited things we say to ourselves in our heads over and over again.

And, as we've been discovering in these pages, our body also talks to itself. Rather than words, our body uses signal messengers called hormones, which are somewhat like the medieval Troubadours who traveled about spreading the news of the kingdom.

Our Inner Troubadours often carry only a single message for a specific organ or system of the body.

Sometimes that message serves us...and sometimes it doesn't. Insulin's job, for example, is to get rid of excess glucose (or sugars) in our bloodstream. If it didn't do this important job we would die. Like, to death and stuff!

So we're not demonizing Insulin here. It's our dutiful pal and we want to maintain a solid relationship with it for those cases where we really need it.

"Insulin is like a broom. It sweeps glucose, amino acids and free fatty acids into cells where potential energy is stored as fat and glycogen to be used later."
--Morrison Bethea, MD, Sam Andrews, MD, Leighton Steward & Luis Balart, MD in *SUGAR BUSTERS!*

However, our sugarized contemporary lifestyles have led us to become virtually *co-dependent on Insulin.* The primary drawback to Insulin is how it accomplishes its mission.

The way this hormone gets rid of our excess glucose is to turn it into fatty acids and store these away as fat—and then act like a prison guard to make sure the newly deposited fat doesn't get back into the bloodstream.

Since the reason you and I are playing this game together is to learn how to effectively lose excess weight, we necessarily want to create an environment within our bodies where Insulin is more of a stranger than a constant companion. That just makes sense, right?!

At the same time, we want to improve our relationship with Glucagon, the dashing hormone that seeks out stored fat, releases it from its cellular prison, and gives it a bus pass for a free ride into our blood supply, where it can finally be burned up as energy.

Remember, the secret to having more Glucagon at our disposal is to cultivate a more moderate blood sugar than most of us are accustomed to. Face it, we're not going to enjoy any of the benefits of Glucagon if we continue on the typical pace of consuming *160 extra pounds of sugar* each year! Just the opposite is true...the fewer excess sugars we consume, the better.

Losing weight is about maintaining a normal blood sugar.

"Take care of your body. It's the only place you have to live."
—Jim Rohn

The Glycemic Index

The Glycemic Index is pretty much the coolest thing ever invented! It was created in the mid-1980's at the University of Toronto to measure how much any particular food we eat raises our blood sugar — which is a really, really, really, really, really (that's 5 "reallys"!) important thing to know.

What's so damn cool about the Glycemic Index (GI) is that it finally gives us a tool to accurately measure how much sugar we are putting into our bloodstream.

The GI uses pure glucose as its primary reference number, assigning it a value of 100.

The closer a food gets to the top of the list, the more it can be compared to pure glucose...which is the form of sugar that humans (and, indeed, all living things) run on.

Foods that contain fewer sugars are assigned a lower number, while foods with more sugars are given a higher number.

One way of looking at the GI is as a useful index of the amount of *damage* any particular food can do to our waistlines. The higher the number on the Glycemic Index, the more Insulin gets "called"...and the lower the number, the less.

And that's really all there is to the Glycemic Index!

How to Use the Glycemic Index

Foods on the Glycemic Index are placed into three categories: High, Medium and Low.

HIGH GI foods rank at **70** or higher on the index
MEDIUM GI foods are **55-70**
LOW GI foods are **55 or LOWER**

When we eat foods with lots of sugars (or, especially, Mega-Sugars, as I refer to them) that rank

HIGH on the GI, our body "calls" more Insulin and we gain more weight.

When we eat foods in the MIDDLE of the GI, we call a little less Insulin and gain slightly less weight.

And when we eat foods LOW on the index, that's when our new BFF Glucagon comes riding in to the rescue to help liberate stored fat, convert it into glucose and burn that shit up! This is the space where we can actually lose weight.

I want to share with you a short list of just a few foods that rank HIGH on the GI, simply to give you idea of what we're dealing with here. I invite you to especially notice where table sugar ranks on this list, and the relative position of some of the foods we commonly think of as "healthy" as compared to raw sugar!

Glucose 100
Russet Potato 98
High Fructose Corn Sugar 90
Instant Rice 90
Popcorn 89
White Rice 83
Pretzels 81
English Muffin 80
Gatorade 80
Waffles 76
Whole Wheat Bread 75
Corn 75
Saltine Crackers 75
White Bread 69
Table Sugar (Sucrose) 59

You may have noticed that raw table sugar is well *below* the list of many popular "healthy" foods that score high on the Glycemic Index.

This means it would actually be preferable (in terms of the amount of Insulin called and the amount of fat we would store) to sit down to a meal where we simply spooned raw sugar into our mouths rather eat a meal of bread, rice, potatoes and other high-GI foods!

Don't get me wrong, eating foods ranking high on the Glycemic Index can be useful...*if* our specific intention is to fatten ourselves up to move to Japan and become professional Sumo wrestlers, lulz!

How High-GI Foods Impact Us

Here's a graphic that neatly shows the effect that eating foods with a high GI has on our bodies...

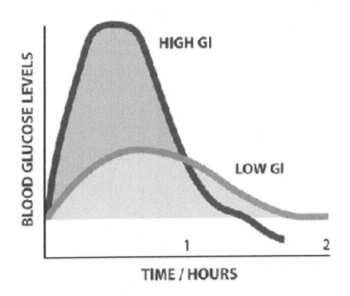

You'll notice that High-GI foods do exactly what we *don't* want, which is spike our blood glucose level.

When that happens, our bodies summon Insulin to gather up all the glucose and stash it away as fat, then make sure it doesn't escape.

But the bad news about going into the red on the

High Glycemic Index doesn't end there. Even worse, about 60 minutes or so after the dramatic rise in glucose caused by High-GI foods comes an equally catastrophic *crash* in the amount of available glucose.

When that happens, our blood sugar level drops *below* the baseline.

Having a normal blood sugar that's riding on top of the baseline is a super-duper good thing because then Glucagon is called to do its fat-liberating heroics. But when our blood sugar level collapses and plunges beneath the baseline, then yet *another* of our Inner Troubadours gets summoned.

This hormone is called **Ghrelin** and it too has but a single message. And that message is to tell our body that we are hungry and it's time to eat again...even though only about an hour or so has passed since we ate a substantial meal!

This is the reason why we can destroy a fully loaded baked potato at lunch and think, "Hey, that should hold us over 'til dinner quite nicely!"

But by the time we get back to the office and sit down at our desk we're already starting to feel hungry again!

Yup, that's the Ghrelin just doing its job.*

(One question unanswerable by the best medical minds of our generation is why the names of so many Hormones sound like minor characters in Shakespearean tragedies. Viz., "Sad-hearted Ghrelin forsoothly into battle on his steady steed did ride!")

The starchy meal we ate at lunch not only spiked our blood sugar and called in mega-doses of Insulin (which means that virtually every bite we took is now being stored as fat), but as our blood sugar roller-coastered back down on the other side it plunged so low that Ghrelin—the Feed-Me-Now Hormone—got called and we're driven to repeat the cycle all over again!

On the other hand, notice in the graphic above that Low GI foods cause a slower, more gentle—and therefore more manageable—rise of glucose in our bloodstream.

Even better, the Low-GI glucose levels descend at an equally leisurely pace and settle nicely right at the baseline.

Eating low on the Glycemic Index doesn't cause us to feel hungry again right away because Ghrelin simply sleeps through the entire affair and is never even woken up to tell us to eat more!

Here's another graphic depiction of the hellish daily roller-coaster ride of living a High-GI lifestyle.

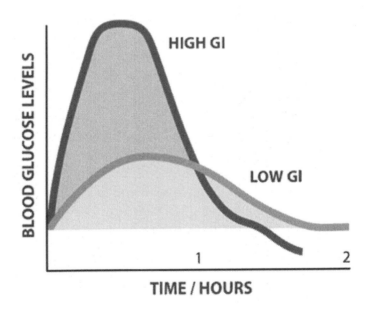

Once again you can see how eating High-GI foods (as we'll discover just ahead, "High-GI" is just shorthand for foods containing lots of sugars and/or Mega-Sugars) causes our blood glucose to spike precipitously and then drop just as drastically below the baseline, which precipitates overwhelming feelings of hunger even though our stomachs are still full from the last meal we ate...leading to more eating, more spiking of our blood sugars, and still more fat being deposited.

A vicious cycle, indeed.

The Glycemic Index and Our Daily Life

The GI score for every food commonly eaten by humankind has already been determined for us by helpful researchers.

While it *is* a very good idea to familiarize ourselves with the GI of the foods we are in the habit of eating frequently, we don't need to make that into any kind of big homework assignment or anything.

Rather than going through all the trouble of memorizing a long list of every High-GI food in the grocery store, we're instead going to follow the example of the indefatigable William Banting.

If you recall, Mr. Banting compiled a very short list of food categories which he referred to as "beans" that he avoided in order to produce his pioneering weight loss.

In the **13 Progressions** that follow, we will assemble our own list of "beans".

I want to assure you in advance that this list of categories of foods to avoid is refreshingly short and easy to sustain as a lifestyle.

It's possible to lump together High-GI foods in just a couple of categories because they all have something in common with one another, just as all the foods that are low on the GI have characteristics in common with each other.

Even so, it's still a good idea to refer to a professionally compiled Glycemic Index from time to time, especially when you're just getting started in creating a revolution in your own life and body.

I don't favor any index over another. There are dozens—if not hundreds—to be found simply by Googling the term "Glycemic Index".

One note of caution: don't get too caught up in the left-brainy task of comparing one list to another. It doesn't really matter if a particular food is 89 on one GI and 86 on another. What matters is that anything in the 80's is well above the minimum threshold of 70 for High GI foods and should be avoided entirely unless you're trying to bulk up to get a college football scholarship or something!

The general rule to follow:

Eat High on the GI (70 or higher) if your goal is to gain lots of weight

Eat Medium on the GI (55-70) if your goal is to gain just a little weight

Eat Low on the GI (0-55) if your goal is to lose belly fat and naturally let go of the pounds

A Quick Word About "Glycemic Load"

If you read any of the excellent books on the proven benefits of eating low on the Glycemic Index that I'll be recommending to you as we go along, sooner or later you'll encounter the concept of "Glycemic Load" (GL).

There's a whole big complicated (well, complicated to *me*, at least!) mathematical equation associated with the Glycemic Load—involving both multiplication *and* division, which is far more math than I prefer to do in an entire year, much less at a single sitting! I personally don't bother with the level of detail involved with working out the Glycemic Load of the foods I consume, but I do want to touch on it briefly.

The general idea behind the Glycemic Load is that you shouldn't just count the sugars or Mega-Sugars in a particular food you eat, but also factor in how much of them you consume.

Of course it's obvious that the more we eat of something, the more we take in of its component nutrients and sugars. In fact, it's so obvious that I don't think we need to mess with the equation of the Glycemic Load, other than understanding it generally.

If one baked potato is bad, then three baked potatoes is worse...we don't need higher math to understand that!

However—and this is more to the point of appreciating Glycemic Load—if we eat a large enough quantity of food from the medium or even the low end of the GI, eventually that too can add up.

Think of it like this...liquor has a much greater alcohol content than beer. Yet if I just have a single shot of tequila I'll be taking in less total alcohol than if I drink an entire 12-pack of beer.

By the same token, even though beer has a relatively low alcohol content, if I do drink a whole dozen of them in one fell swoop then I'll become more intoxicated than I would by downing simply that single shot of tequila. Ya dig?!

Virtually all fruits and all vegetables score low on the GI. However, none of them score a 0 and the vast majority have a rating somewhere in the 5-30 range.

That means it is certainly possible to build up an *overall* high Glycemic Load even if we consume only fruits and vegetables so long as we eat enough of them.

Primates like gorillas eat a pure vegetarian diet, but

because of their overall Glycemic Load they end up with large, protruding bellies.

It is possible to live a *Low Carb Revolution* lifestyle as a vegetarian, but that is a more difficult task. I'm going to give you some specific tips later to help you accomplish that if your heart is set on being a vegetarian.

But first…coming up next we're going to learn some fascinating distinctions about why we become hungry, when we know we're full…and how to curb our appetite naturally, from the inside out! Sound like fun?!

"The major studies show that there is hardly anything in common among those who reach 100 years of age. They have high cholesterol and low cholesterol. Some exercise and some don't. Some smoke and some don't. Some are nasty as can be, and some nice and calm. However, they all have low sugar, low triglycerides, and low Insulin relative to their age. If there is a single marker for lifespan it is Insulin…and the way to treat all the so-called chronic diseases of aging is to treat Insulin levels."
— Ron Rosedale, MD

KEY #9:
"How to Feel Less Hungry"

Let's Have an Affair

I want you to have an affair! Before you get your panties all in a knot, allow me to explain. I don't want you to have an actual affair. (I mean, have one or don't have one, it doesn't matter to me. Do whatever works for you!)

No, what I'm talking about here is having an affair on the *inside* of you.

Back when I weighed close to 270 pounds I was hungry all the time. The more I ate and the more I weighed, the hungrier I got.

You might have had a similar experience in your own life. You're eating all the time and yet still feel hungry...all the damn time!

Now why is that?! *Why* do we feel hungrier and hungrier as we gain more weight?

We're about to discover exactly why that happens. Along the way we'll meet the next of our Inner Troubadours who play a role in the unfolding saga of assisting us to release the excess weight and belly fat we've been carrying around.

If we are currently overweight it's because we've been stepping out with the hormone Insulin way too much for our own good.

Insulin has been imprisoning the excess glucose in our bloodstream as fat and then guarding it so that it can't escape.

At the heart of the *Low Carb Revolution* is renewing our relationship with the debonair hormone Glucagon, which rides gallantly in to the rescue and frees the trapped fat in our cells so it can be burned up as energy.

If our goal is to no longer gain any additional weight, then having a nice relationship with Glucagon is crucial. Indeed, if our goal is to *lose* weight, then we want to be as monogamous with Glucagon as possible...and that means eating low on the Glycemic Index.

The more we consume Low to No GI foods (and yes, there are actually tons and tons of foods that rank 0 on the Glycemic Index, meaning we can eat them in virtually unlimited quantities and still lose weight), the more "faithful" we will be to our new paramour, Glucagon.

As a natural byproduct of this lifestyle, we will necessarily also be "calling" yet another one of our Inner Troubadours. So we're going to have an affair, if you will, with a very special hormone.

Meet Leptin

The name of our little something-something on the side here is Leptin...who also follows the by-now-predictable pattern of sounding like its name was lifted directly from a play by Mr. William Shakespeare. ("Fair Leptin hath for thirty days, and an equal number of nights, run amok!")

Anyway, Leptin, what the heck is that?! Leptin is the Troubadour who carries the rather significant message to our bodies that says, "Stop eating—you're full!"

The hormone Leptin signals to our brains that our body has had enough to eat, producing the much-desired sensation of satiety...a sensation, by the way, that folks on those sad calorie-restricted diets never,

ever get to enjoy until the inevitable day when they dump their wretched food scale in the rubbish bin and get back to living!

Although researchers have known for a loooooong time that we had some kind of mechanism in our body to tell us when to quit eating, Leptin was only isolated and identified as recently as 1995.

Leptin is our innate, natural appetite suppressant. That's a good thing, right?! Suppressing our appetite is something we all probably want a little more of if our goal is to lose our nasty belly fat and return to our natural state and birthright of our Ideal Body, wouldn't you say?

However, the way Leptin is "called" by our body is, at first glance, counter-intuitive...although when I explain the evolutionary reason behind it, everything will make perfect sense. (Now I don't mean *everything* in the world will make perfect sense, of course, just everything to do with why you sometimes feel hungry no matter how much you've already eaten will make sense!)

More Fat = "Less" Leptin

So we might imagine that if we are overweight and have all this fat stored up in our body that Leptin would be running around hither and yon suppressing our appetite so we could finally burn off all the energy that Insulin had so carefully imprisoned in our cells. But it doesn't work that way.

The level of circulating Leptin within our bodies is directly proportional to the amount of fat we have stored.

The more we weigh, the more Leptin we have, BUT...the weaker and less effective it is.

We become desensitized to the Leptin, so the net result is that our bodies behave like we now have less

Leptin available.

Let's hit the rewind button on this one, since this point is vital: The amount of the hormone that tells us to stop eating *effectively* goes down as our weight goes up!

Although, again, in a purely scientific sense, the amount of Leptin doesn't actually go *down*, it certainly seems that way inside our bloodstreams because the high quantities of stored fat cause us to become increasingly resistant to Leptin's effects.

So...the more fat stored in our bodies, the less effective Leptin is at telling at our tell our stomachs to stop feeling hunger.

I know, I know, totally unfair, right?!

The reason for this has to do with our old "friend" (and with friends like this, who needs enemies, badda-boom!) Insulin.

Excessive amounts of Insulin in our bodies—which, as you recall, is the inevitable result of eating high on the Glycemic Index—actually inhibits Leptin and keeps it from being "called" in to share its message.

Here's how it all plays out inside us...

Bob and Leptin Have a Falling Out

My friend Bob is a funny, funny man (and a bit of a name-dropper, I should add!) He's a talented character actor and a popular teacher of improvisational comedy in Austin, TX.

Like many other funny people before him, Bob is a bit heavy and he's quite keen on becoming, well, not so heavy.

Left to his own devices, Bob does what virtually all Americans are taught to do—which is to eat as meagerly as humanly possible, and then do enough physical activity each day to burn off the precious few calories he allows to pass his lips.

For breakfast, Bob "restricts" himself to merely a chai latte and a single bagel from an anonymous Carbo-Centric business whose name rhymes with "Glar-glucks".

A little tea with milk ("chai" is just hipster-speak for spiced tea and milk!) and a single bagel...doesn't seem like much, does it? Bob no doubt feels he's starting off his day with a healthy dose of "suffering for his waistline" by consuming such a modest amount of calories for breakfast.

Unlike Bob, you and I know that calories have *nothing* whatsoever to do with gaining weight or losing weight. It's the sugars and Mega-Sugars (carbohydrates) that count.

Well, Bob's Venti chai has a staggering 72 grams of carbohydrates, and there's another 50 grams of carbs in the bagel—and that's before Bob tipples additional sugar into his drink and then loads up the bagel with cream cheese, jelly and other sugary toppings.

In other words, my friend Bob is the Sir Edmund Hillary of the Glycemic Index, charting new heights that no man has ever ascended before—all in the name of a "healthy" breakfast!

The Glycemic Index is ultimately a measure of the amount of carbohydrates in the foods we eat and the drinks we drink. The more carbohydrates (which I often refer to by their more accurate name of "Mega-Sugars) we consume, the higher our glucose levels rise and the more fat our inner Troubadour called Insulin is forced to store and guard.

"The natural healing force within us is the greatest force in getting well."
--Hippocrates

Exceeding Carrying Capacity!

Starbucks has introduced a new, larger size called the Trenta. The Trenta holds 916 milliliters of liquid Carbohydrates. Yet the human stomach can only hold 900 ml--meaning this single beverage will exceed the carrying capacity of our entire stomach!

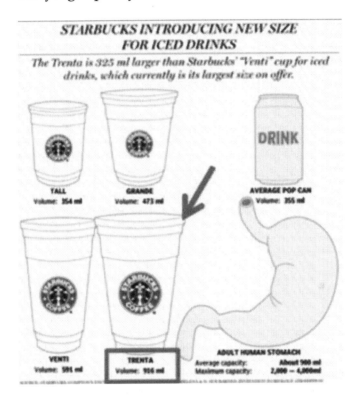

This is a quite formidable enemy we're going up against! They have deep pockets and a vested interest in keeping us fat, content and asleep.

A Comedy of Errors

Since my friend Bob knows quite a bit more about comedy than about nutrition, he's actually quite proud of himself this morning for his "prudent" eating habits.

He believes he's started off his day with a "light" snack that will contribute to his desired weight loss, whereas, in point of fact, the chai and bagel score near the top of the GI and are now wreaking havoc on the glucose levels in his bloodstream.

As Bob's glucose levels soar, Insulin pours into his bloodstream in a desperate attempt to convert all that glucose into fatty acids that can be locked up in his cells.

Meanwhile, his Inner Troubadour called Leptin is getting ready to make its rounds and deliver its message telling Bob to stop eating because he's now full.

But it turns out that Insulin is a jealous little bitch! Insulin doesn't want any other hormones running around talking to the stomach and stuff...so Insulin basically hits Leptin over the head with a club and drags its rival Troubadour into a dark alley and leaves it there.

By the time Leptin recovers consciousness, it's too late to deliver its message—Bob is already starting to feel hungry again, and is trying to justify grabbing some waffles on his way to teaching his first comedy class of the day. (For some reason comedians are ALWAYS eating waffles. They just like everything about waffles—from the name, to their unique, indented pattern and even their Frisbee-like capacity to be launched into the audience! Seriously, if you ever want to befriend a comic, just buy her a box of frozen waffles and she'll follow you around like a puppy for a week!)

Okay, so the more Insulin Bob has in his bloodstream from eating a "light" breakfast that scores near the top of the Glycemic Index, the more fat Bob will store in his body... and yet the less effective Leptin will be at telling his stomach to stop feeling hungry!

Another vicious cycle, no?! Truly the rich get richer and the poor (those of us who are overweight) get poorer. But, not to worry, we've got a plan here!

Why is Bob Overweight...and Tired All the Time?

My funny friend Bob will never tire of reminding you that he knows a lot of semi-famous actors and comedians—people whose names you would kinda-sorta know, whose late-night Comedy Central specials you might stumble upon, whose voices you would vaguely recognize once they started talking.

But, like most people, Bob doesn't know his own body very well at all.

If you were to ask Bob why he's overweight, he would probably say it's because he eats too many calories and burns too few calories through exercise—which is, of course, the same, tired Calorie Myth of Weight Gain that's been pounded into every last man Jack of us our entire lives.

Unlike Bob, you and I know the reason he stores fat in his body is because he's living high on the Glycemic Index—consuming carb-filled foods and drinks like chai lattes and bagels.

Besides eating and drinking the wrong things, Bob does also probably eat and drink too much of them. That's because all the Insulin flooding his blood stream inhibits the release of our natural appetite suppressant hormone Leptin.

And the less Leptin that Bob has at his disposal, the hungrier he feels during all hours of the day and night. This soon becomes a self-perpetuating cycle.

As a result, Bob is NOT overweight because he eats too much food. Instead, he eats too much food BECAUSE he's overweight.

We don't become overweight because we eat too much food.
We eat too much food because we are overweight.

I know this is exactly the *opposite* of what you've been told your entire life...but so, too, is almost everything I'll be sharing with you throughout this entire book!

Obesity is caused by excess fat accumulation...not by eating too many calories or getting too little exercise.

Being overweight and inactive are the SYMPTOMS of obesity, not the CAUSE. Does that make sense? We don't get fat because we overeat; we overeat because our cells have accumulated excess fat, which is whole different kettle of fish!

As we've already learned, feeling hungry all the time is the fault of Leptin...or, more precisely, the effective lack of Leptin in our system because it's being blocked by the overwhelming Insulin load from all the Mega-Sugars we consume with almost religious intensity.

All the hormones we've been talking about naturally have little secret talents and hobbies on the side.

In the case of Leptin, besides carrying the important message of satiety and fullness, it also happens to regulate *all* aspects of Energy Metabolism. As neurosurgeon and low-carbohydrate activist Jack Kruse, MD, puts it: "Leptin controls the machinery of energy generation for humans. It is like our photosynthesis."

Bob is currently heavy, which means he's already *effectively* got less circulating Leptin available to him because of the high-carb, high-sugar, high-Insulin lifestyle that made him heavy in the first place.

And the less Leptin at his disposal, the less overall

energy Bob has to draw upon in his life. (Which also answers the rhetorical question Bob so often poses in his Facebook status, "Why am I so tired all the time?")

Dr. J. Fred Andrews of Trinity College, Dublin describes the actions of Leptin as being like a "quartermaster" that regulates the energy levels available to all our bodily systems, while Jack Kruse, MD, ups the ante by maintaining that Leptin has as profound a role on our metabolism and available energy as the Sun itself does for all of the natural world.

> *"What would happen to life on earth if we eliminated all coal, oil, nuclear fuel and sunlight from our planet? Life would be changed dramatically and quickly. When Leptin is not working correctly, this is precisely the fate our cells have to deal with and it can dramatically alter how our cells or organ systems respond when fuel demands cannot keep pace with needs."*
> — Dr. Jack Kruse

How to Have An Affair With Leptin

This is the really fun and really easy part of the *Low Carb Revolution*! You already know there's nothing in this lifestyle about counting calories or portion controls.

At the same time, it would be nice to at least have the option to eat a little bit less rather than be possessed by a constant, overwhelming urge from within telling us to eat more and more and more, wouldn't you agree?!

We now know that the hormone Leptin is the secret behind having the option to eat less...to stop feeling hungry even after a relatively modest meal compared to what it previously took to sate us.

Not only do increased levels of circulating Leptin

keep us feeling full, but that very same Leptin also helps give us the necessary energy to get off our butts and go outside to play more!

And the only thing we have to do to get down and dirty with Leptin at each meal is what we were already gonna do — which is eat Low on the Glycemic Index!

Remember, the less Insulin that gets called when we eat a meal, the more Leptin we have at our disposal…and this is the Troubadour bearing the good news, "All is full in the kingdom of your stomach — cease all eating activities henceforth!"

By eating a Low-GI meal, we start feeling full faster and we stay feeling full longer.

If my friend Bob (have I mentioned lately how *funny* Bob is?!) were to avoid sugars and carbohydrates in the mornings, his blood glucose would stay low, the amount of Insulin in his system would be negligible, and before you know it his long-lost friend Leptin would show up and instruct Bob to stop eating forthwith.

Only when we eat medium or high on the Glycemic Index do we feel compelled to continue eating more and more because we effectively have no Leptin to tell our bodies otherwise.

Ugh, Can't We Just Make A Shot for This?!

Much to the chagrin of Big Pharmacy, giving subjects (that's how they think of us, as *subjects*) external doses of Leptin does NOT work well in suppressing our appetites.

Well, it does work, sort of…but the *quantity* we have to be injected with is so high that the Leptin would seriously have to be shipped in gallon jugs rather than tiny vials.

And the heavier we are, the more Leptin we would need to make the slightest difference in our systems.

Plus, if the "subjects" are still living a high-GI/high-Insulin lifestyle (which most of them are, naturally) the added Leptin won't have any lasting effect in any case.

So much for better living through chemistry!

Okay, so what is going on here, anyway? Why should we effectively have less Leptin the heavier we grow?

It certainly seems as if a body that has gained too much weight should have the good sense to say, "Hey, fat-ass, step away from the fattening carbohydrates, you've had enough to eat for now!" instead of sending the exact opposite message and encouraging us to eat still more.

Why in the world would our bodies tell us to continue eating when we're already gaining too much weight and producing more than an average amount of Insulin?!

Big Pharmacy is frankly clueless about the answer, because they don't view their subjects (i.e., us) as whole, complicated systems that interact with the larger world around us.

Instead they see us a bio-mechanical collection of smaller parts and sub-systems, each of which supposedly operates independently of the others in the same way that the brakes of your car have nothing to do with the machinery that controls your windshield wipers or turn-signals.

Big Pharmacy remains confused about why they can't figure out how come injecting more and more Leptin into over-sized subjects doesn't help suppress their over-sized appetites...and so they just continue throwing away hundreds of millions of research dollars every year trying to figure it out.

But you're in luck, my friend. I'm going to solve the problem for you right here, right now, and for no additional charge!

I'm about to explain to you *why* gaining weight actually causes us to feel more hungry and leads us to overeat even more. And, of course, then I'm going to let you know specifically what *you* can do to turn that completely around in your own body.

How We Ate For Most of History

For most of the first two million years of human evolution we had no refrigeration, no Tupperware, no zip-lock bags...and therefore no way to preserve the food we caught or found for leaner times.

We ate whatever food we had before it spoiled. When all the food we had was gone or spoiled, we starved until we could find more.

For approximately 1.99 million years of our history, food was plentiful in the spring, summer and fall, so we ate as much as possible.

During the winter, food was scarce and we had far less to eat. It soon developed that an excellent evolutionary strategy would be to somehow plan ahead for the lean times and *store* some food in advance.

Since, again, there was no way to preserve food for extended periods of time, the only place to "store" it was inside of us...in our bellies, for example.

To be sure, some early humans disagreed with this new strategy.

They ate just a "normal amount" during times of plenty, and many of them ended up starving to death during the lean winter months. We have a name for these early humans: *extinct*!

Meanwhile, other early humans—our forefathers and foremothers—figured out that if they ate a little more even when there was still plenty of food, then they would have reserves within themselves to make it through winter.

This strategy of over-eating during times of plenty

so we could survive during the inevitable annual cycle of not-so-plenty worked out fantastically. The early humans who devised it lived long enough to reproduce and, little by little, all existing humans evolved to have this survival strategy built into our very physiology.

And the strategy goes something like this...when there is an abundance of food, we are driven to eat more of it to prepare ourselves for the famine that will surely follow.

So every fall, when food was still plentiful, early humans would overeat and gain bellies — thus storing up potential energy for winter.

Since they hadn't yet invented calendars or bank holidays or Thanksgiving, their only signal that lean times were coming was that abundant times were already *here*.

It's not just humans who do this, of course. Bears and other hibernating mammals famously gain weight during times of feast in order to survive the ensuing times of wintery famine.

In both bears and humans, when more Insulin is circulating in the blood from all the feasting, the less Leptin there is to tell them to stop eating.

It's vitally important to understand that it's *not* lack of will-power or self-control that causes us to overeat and always feel hungry when we become heavy and filled with Insulin, that's just how we evolved.

A Never-Ending Land of Plenty

Less than a thousand years ago, which is just a blink of an eye in evolutionary terms, we finally discovered the first primitive methods to preserve food from times of abundance to see us through times of lack-osity. Humans originally preserved food by packing it in salt, curing it, drying it out, etc., which was a good start.

And it's been less than a century since we figured

out refrigeration, which allowed long-term storage of all kinds of foods on a widespread basis.

Nowadays, of course, we can go to the grocery store and buy enough food for a week or even several months and refrigerate/freeze it until we're ready to eat it.

We live in a world where it's now always feast. As long as we have the means, there's always plenty of food to be had.

You and I know that. But our bodies don't. A generation spans about 20 years. We've experienced a scant 5 generations of evolution in the century since the early methods of refrigeration and the now-ubiquitous grocery stores created our never-ending, all-you-can-eat buffet.

Meanwhile, we have 99,995 (give or take a handful!) generations of human evolution under our belts that created an internal environment where the mere *presence* of the fat-storage hormone Insulin in our bloodstream deliberately blocked the appetite-suppressant Leptin.

In the past, whenever we started to eat more and get fat and have more Insulin in our system, our body figured (rightly, it turned out) that famine was fast approaching.

And rather than have stupid old Leptin undo all its hard work of fattening up for lean times by telling us to stop eating, the body figured out how to use Insulin to club Leptin over the head and dump it in a dark alley.

Therefore we have a genetic memory of close to 100,000 generations of our forefathers and foremothers overeating during at least one part of the year in order to survive until spring.

And Now For The Good News

The good news in all this is that you and I have science

on our side.

We don't need no stinkin' shots of manufactured Leptin because we now know exactly what to do in order to never trigger our body's Winter's Coming So Hurry Up And Eat As Much As Possible strategy.

And that is to *simply eat low on the Glycemic Index!* Once again, the lower we eat on the GI, the less Insulin we'll have in our system; the less fat-storing Insulin, the more fat-releasing Glucagon and the more appetite-suppressing, energy-giving Leptin we get to enjoy.

It's a win-win-win situation for us and our beautiful bodies to live a Low-GI lifestyle!

Okay, it's high time you and I take a brief, yet profoundly important, detour into a topic we haven't explored much yet. This topic is really the elephant in the room at the foundation of everything we'll be achieving together in this book.

Let's talk...carbs.

> *"I saw only a few die of hunger--of over-eating, a hundred thousand."*
> — Ben Franklin

KEY #10:
"The Truth About Carbohydrates"

Sugar Is Not Food

First, the bad news...we don't need sugars to live. In no way, shape or form are sugars required in our diet in order for us to live a long, happy, healthy, productive lifestyle.

Recall that humans of one variety or another have been around for some 2 million years and, up until quite recently, there was little or no sugar to be found.

Crystallized sugar as we know it today wasn't even invented until the end of the 5th Century in India...where all kinds of other cool things were also going down.

If you'd been alive back in the year 500 AD, India was definitely the happening spot in the world.

For one thing, India was enjoying a Golden Age of Mathematics, a series of stunningly original scholars were creating mathematical concepts that would haunt high school juniors and seniors to this very day.

Just a very few of the mathematical discoveries of that era...

The roots of modern trigonometry
Quadratic equations
Accurate calculations for solar and lunar eclipses
The value of pi to 4 decimal places

But it was another discovery in that same brief period that would later go on to change the world even more profoundly.

Around the year 502, an unsung Indian merchant who traded in sugarcane juice discovered how to crystallize the liquid into "refined" sugar — thus making the sweet juice less bulky and cumbersome to transport, as well as longer-lasting.

And thus crystallized sugar was born. Of course, it's not like it was an overnight success or anything.

"How Sweet it is!"

In those dark days before Al Gore invented the Internet, it took a looooong time for new ideas to spread...centuries, in fact.

It wasn't until more than 500 years later, during the Crusades, that crystallized sugar was first introduced to Europe and the Western world.

Even during the Middle Ages and right up until the beginning of the Victorian Era, only royalty and the fanciest people could afford to taste sugar in their entire lives.

Fast forward all the way to the dawn of the 20th Century. As we learned earlier, as recently as 1900 Americans consumed an average of only about one pound of added sugar in an entire year, compared to the staggering 160 lbs. of excess sugars foisted on Americans today by Big Food.

So our obsession with sugar is brand-new in evolutionary terms. We didn't evolve as a species to process excess sugars in our bloodstreams.

For the first couple million years of being here, during which we had access to little or no sugar, we flourished just fine.

Sugar is not a required or necessary part of the human diet. Tasty, yes...needed to sustain life, nope.

Sweet Nothingness

Sugar was sparingly used for most of recorded US

history. The memorable accomplishments of previous generations of Americans were achieved on a diet of less sugar in a lifetime than the average American now ingests every month!

Again, I'm not suggesting that sugar isn't fun or yummy — it most certainly is! We just need to understand that sugar isn't any kind of essential nutrient or anything.

In fact, sugar contains no nutrients of any kind. I mean, there's never gonna be a minimum Recommended Daily Allowance (RDA) for sugar!

Sugar contains no protein, no vitamins, no minerals, no nothing. 1 gram of sugar also equals 1 gram of carbohydrates...because sugars and carbohydrates are the same thing. Well, to be more precise, sugars are a category of carbohydrates.

Carbohydrates Are Sugars

Raw table sugar is a simple carbohydrate, with anywhere from one to a dozen or more sugar molecules strung together. We refer to these as Simple Sugars or just Sugars.

Next up comes the category most of us conjure up when we think about "carbohydrates" or "high-carb", and these are the Complex Sugars with hundreds of different sugar molecules strung together, which I jokingly refer to as Mega-Sugars, since that's what they truly are.

Finally come the Mega-Mega-Sugars — more popularly known as Starches.

Simple Sugars (table sugar) fall close to the middle of the Glycemic Index at about 59.

Traditional carbohydrates (Mega-Sugars) like bread and other wheat products score high on the GI — in the 70s and 80s.

Starches (Mega-Mega-Sugars) like corn starch, rice

starch, potatoes and other starchy, root vegetables rank at the very tippy top of the GI — virtually nothing scores higher other than straight glucose!

Eating High on the GI

Remember earlier when we learned all about the Glycemic Index and how foods with a high GI call in the hormone Insulin, which causes us to store fat in our bodies and pack on the pounds? Those were good times, right?!

One question we didn't ask then, but we will now, is *why* certain foods rank high on the Glycemic Index and others rank low?

As we've just seen…it's the sugars, baby. The more sugars a food possesses — progressing from simple sugars to complex sugars to starches — the higher the ranking.

100% of the top spots on the GI are held by carbohydrates, with the worst offenders being the super-carbohydrates called starches. *The Glycemic Index, then, is based entirely on how many carbohydrates a food contains.* If a food or drink contains just a few carbs , it will summon a smallish amount of our fat-storing Troubadour known as Insulin and cause us to gain a smallish amount of weight.

If a food contains a larger amount of the complex sugars known as carbohydrates, then the GI number grows higher still, and the more Insulin gets called and the more weight we gain.

And if a food or drink is made up of starches, then the GI is almost off the chart and our Insulin is gonna be working overtime storing fat within us!

Most of us have grown up hearing the message over and over again that not only are carbohydrates good for us, but they're an important component of our daily nutritional intake. I'd like to suggest to you that there's a word for this dietary advice. It's not, let's politely say, *true*.

Carbohydrates are nothing more and nothing less than long-chain sugar molecules. Carbohydrates are not food and they are not necessary for human life.

They are simply an amped-up version of regular sugar and are more properly referred to as Mega-Sugars.

> *"There are only two mistakes one can make along the road to truth: not going all the way and not starting."*
> —Buddha

KEY #11:
"Attack of the Mega-Sugars"

What Are Mega-Sugars?

For reasons we'll explore in just a bit, in the United States we've been told for the past twenty years that the majority of our daily intake of calories should come from carbohydrates.

We've been instructed by glossy magazines filled with glossy ads for sports drinks that we absolutely need to do something called "carb-loading" before the Big Race and we need to "replenish" our carbs every time we break a sweat.

So we've dutifully become carb-aholics, even though the average person on the street doesn't have the slightest understanding of what a carbohydrate is in the first place.

And why should they? The term "carbohydrate" doesn't give us any particularly useful information about what they are.

But it turns out there's an *alternate* name for carbohydrates, and this is the name used most commonly in scientific circles.

Researchers regularly refer to carbohydrates by its scientific name of saccharides. (Indeed, if you type "saccharide" into Google, the very first result will be the Wikipedia article on "carbohydrates, aka, saccharides", because these are just two names for the exact same thing.)

Saccharide comes from the Greek word *sakchar*,

meaning sugar or sweetness, which tells us all we need to know about what carbohydrates/saccharides really are.

Formally, carbohydrates/saccharides are sugar chains...groups of complex sugars all strung together.

Once we know that the synonym for carbohydrates is saccharides and we also understand that they are simply made up of sugar chains, then we can start putting carbohydrates/saccharides into their proper place in our daily intake of food.

To help us do that, I've coined the cheeky moniker of Mega-Sugars to refer to carbohydrates/saccharides. Mega meaning a "bunch"...and sugar meaning, well, "sugar".

Basically, Mega-Sugars (carbohydrates) are like regular sugars on steroids. If we eat a sugary food, it summons our hard-working Troubadour called Insulin to come do its job of storing fat for a rainy day that never comes.

If we eat a food high in Mega-Sugars, it pushes Insulin almost to its limit.

Let's take another glance at our list of some representative High GI foods from earlier. Note that foods scoring high on the Glycemic Index all have one thing in common: their excessive carbohydrate count.

Glucose 100
Russet Potato 98
High Fructose Corn Sugar 90
Instant Rice 90
Popcorn 89
White Rice 83
Pretzels 81
English Muffin 80
Gatorade 80
Waffles 76

Whole Wheat Bread 75
Corn 75
Saltine Crackers 75
White Bread 69
Table Sugar (Sucrose) 59

The Devil Amongst Us

Over the past few years, High Fructose Corn Syrup (HFCS) been demonized--and quite rightly so. But why exactly is HFCS the declared enemy of our health and waistlines?! What's in it that's so damn bad for us?

It turns out that out of every 100 grams of HFCS, 76 of them are Mega-Sugars!

The stuff is just liquid carbohydrates, which is why it scores an astronomical 90 on the GI. Still, the most common source of Mega-Sugars in the SAD (Standard American Diet) come from grains, breads, cereals and pastas, which fall under the overall category of "Wheat Products".

Since Wheat Products are comprised primarily of Mega-Sugars, they uniformly rank high on the GI, well above even raw sugar itself. (After all, that's why they're called *Mega*-Sugars, because the effect they have on our bodies is mega-worse than "mere" sugar.) Keep in mind that the *taste* of a food has no particular relationship to how much of the fat-storing hormone Insulin it produces.

We would probably imagine that eating a bowl of chocolate and vanilla ice cream swirled together would go straight to our thighs.

However, we probably wouldn't imagine that eating a bowl of plain pasta — which tastes bland rather than sweet — is actually far *worse* for us than the ice cream, in terms of ranking high on the Glycemic Index and calling greater amounts of fat-storing Insulin into our bloodstream.

"Wheat products elevate our blood sugar levels more than virtually any other carbohydrate, from beans to candy bars. This has important implications for body weight, since glucose is unavoidably accompanied by Insulin, the hormone that allows entry of glucose into the cells of the body, converting the glucose to fat. The higher the glucose after consumption of food, the greater the Insulin level, the more fat is deposited."
— William Davis, MD

Carbohydrates = Mega-Sugars

Let's be perfectly clear about all this. We discussed the mechanisms of storing fat in our bodies through Insulin and the advantages of creating an inner environment of less Insulin if our goal is to lose weight.

And we learned how to begin cultivating a new relationship with our fat-liberating hero, Glucagon, by eating in such a way that our bloodstream enjoys lower, more manageable levels of glucose.

To achieve this end, we explored the benefits of consulting the Glycemic Index, which tells us exactly which foods summon Insulin (those that score high on the GI) and which foods summon Glucagon (those that score low.) And we've now found out that the *reason* foods rank high on the GI is because they contain more carbohydrates (which is just Orwellian double-speak for what they really are, Mega-Sugars) and the reason other foods rank low on the GI is because they contain fewer sugars.

In a phrase....*if our goal is to lose weight, sugars are bad...while carbohydrates (Mega-Sugars) are even badder.*

Is this making sense? In the next chapter we're going to "check our work", as they used to say in school.

Before we go any further, we're going to compare

what we've learned against observable aspects of American culture to make sure all this fits together into a complete, coherent model of how we can finally lose weight and keep it off forever.

So What *Do* We Need to Stay Alive?

Oh, by the way, despite what "they" keep telling us, we do *not* need sugars or carbohydrates to live. They add nothing to the dance of life. Absolutely nothing!

Again, I'm not saying that sugars and other carbs don't taste good or provide a scrumptious treat for our tongues, I just want you to grasp the concept that they are not needed to sustain life.

We don't need added sugars or added carbohydrates to live and thrive as humans. In fact, the less we have of both, the better our lives will be in every way, shape and form.

So what DO we need to live full, happy and healthy lives? Not counting water and air and hugs, of course, what specific types of foods *must* we take in to keep our bodies going?

Well it turns out there are only 3 major specific categories that humans require for survival:

Protein to rebuild our cells—which are themselves largely protein and water

Fat to supply us with the energy to leap tall buildings in a single bound

Fiber (or roughage) to help absorb water and flush out waste products

That's it. Just those three things—protein, fat and fiber. Notice what's *not* on that list....

Carbohydrates/sacchrides are not on the list, because ingesting external sources of sugars and Mega-Sugars is *not* necessary to human life...it's only necessary if our goal is to create human fat!

We need **Protein** to rebuild the 65 trillion cells that make up our bodies.

We need **Fat** to supply the energy or calories to power an energetic, productive lifestyle.

And we need **Fiber** to serve as roughage and scour the decks, if you will.

Fiber is really a special category all by itself, and not a macronutrient like protein and fat. Fiber occurs naturally in all plant foods—fruits, vegetables, beans, nuts and seeds, doesn't matter. (Meanwhile, animal foods like meats, fish and dairy products have no fiber to speak of—which is a big reason why we couldn't subsist on eating meat alone.)

Although fiber is technically a carbohydrate, by definition fiber is largely indigestible and so it doesn't have the same fat-creating impact on our bloodstreams as do true Mega-Sugars like bread and pasta.

When people tell us we "need" carbohydrates to live, what they really mean is that we need the very specific type of carbohydrate called Fiber in order to live. But, again, we get that naturally in this cool thing they invented called "food".

We don't require any other carbohydrate besides Fiber in our diets.

"Carbohydrates are not necessary building blocks of other molecules. The body can obtain all its energy from protein and fat."
—Wikipedia article on "Carbohydrates"

But...But Elite Athletes Do It

If you've seen one or more Gatorade ads in your life, then all this might be a tough sell for you because they've got you convinced to the core of your being that even if the Mega-Sugars that we call carbohydrates aren't necessary for life, they sure as hell are necessary in order to win the Big Race!

Hey…now might be a good time to remind you that Gatorade is owned by PepsiCo, the $60 billion a year pillar of Big Food built entirely on selling carbohydrates in the form of liquids (Gatorade, 7-Up, Mountain Dew, Pepsi, etc.) and carbohydrates in the form of solids (Lay's, Doritos and Quaker Oats, etc.)

So the very organization "helpfully" teaching us that it's healthy and necessary to eat and drink more carbohydrates in the first place is the very same one selling us these products! Seriously?!

Even so, let's do chat about the idea that athletes need added carbohydrates, because there *is* something to this notion.

Immediate vs. Sustained Energy Needs

Again, all plant foods contain natural carbohydrates, mostly in the form of Fiber. Beyond eating plenty of fruits and vegetables, we never need to ingest a single added carbohydrate in our entire lives!

Now glucose is the fuel our body uses to power us in everything we do and carbohydrates *are* an immediate source of glucose—which is quite useful if, say, we're bicycling straight up a mountain in the Tour de France.

But in 99.999% of the situations in which we will find ourselves in our entire lives, our immediate energy needs are unlikely to be so dire that we must rely on extra carbohydrates to meet them.

The average person stores about 1500 grams of glycogen—enough to run about 20 miles at a full tilt. (This is why marathoners so often bonk at the 20-mile mark in their races...it took that long to deplete energy they had stored for ready access in their bodies!)

So right now, sitting there reading this, you've got approximately enough energy stored up within you to run a good 20 miles...which is, I'm proud to say, is about 10 miles more than the grand *total* of all the miles I've run in my entire life! (More on why I'm not a fan of running for health *or* weight-loss reasons in Part Two.)

In most ordinary situations, we don't so much need an *immediate* source of glucose as we do a *sustained* source of it.

And a sustained source of energy comes from the protein and fat in meats, fish, poultry, seeds, nuts and even vegetables.

Our body uses the amino acids in these foods to create glucose to supply our energy needs.

> *"Amino acids can be converted into glucose by the liver through a process called gluconeogenesis, which is the manufacture of glucose from noncarbohydrate food sources, such as protein. The body's ability to manufacture its own glucose is important for maintaining normal energy requirements."*
> — Morrison Bethea, MD, Sam Andrews, MD, Leighton Steward & Luis Balart, MD in *SUGAR BUSTERS!*

Energy to Spare

I live an exceedingly active lifestyle. I regularly walk, bicycle, and/or swim for at least an hour every single day and, in addition to that, I go dancing 5-7 times per week, often for 2-3 hours at a time.

My high energy needs are more than adequately met through the fat and protein I consume naturally from a variety of meat, fish and poultry products, as well as an unlimited diet of all the vegetables and fruits I desire. No matter how strenuous my play, at no time do I need or require any added carbohydrates in order to enjoy all the energy (and more) I need to sustain my active lifestyle 365 days per year.

But any fool can run around with lots of energy. Even more importantly, I enjoy what I refer to as abundant vitality. By "vitality" I mean the ability to sit down and focus my entire body and mind on a task at hand for as long as required in order to accomplish it.

Accessing our inner vitality to compose a symphony or write a book requires not just an abundance of energy, but an abundance of *clarity*—a clarity not readily available to people still stuck on the high-carb hampster wheel.

As an example of the vitality endlessly available to me without any added carbohydrates, as I type this very sentence I have been sitting here writing steadily on the *Low Carb Revolution* for the last 3 hours and 38 minutes with only two of brief bathroom breaks.

Back when I consumed a typical High-Carb diet (also known as SAD, or the Standard American Diet) it took all the effort I could summon to sit still for even 15-20 minutes of writing or thinking. Carbohydrates can only give us energy in short, quickly fading bursts, not over the long haul that it takes to accomplish anything meaningful in life.

> *"The food you eat can be either the safest and most powerful form of medicine, or the slowest form of poison."*
> — Dr. Ann Wigmore

Carbohydrates *Are* a Quick Source of Energy

However, there are times in our lives when our immediate energy needs can outstrip the easily available supply...when we need a little "lighter fluid", if you will, to jump start the blaze within us. In those circumstances, fruits are the best source of immediate, natural energy: they taste good, they're good for us,

121

and they can be eaten in pretty much unlimited quantities.

Besides being a quick energy source, fruits (like all plant foods) are also rich in vitamins, minerals and phytochemicals — profoundly important micronutrients that positively affect our health, but which occur in such diminutive quantities that they haven't yet been established as essential nutrients by whomever it is who decides these things.

While the number of known vitamins and minerals number in the dozens, so far researchers have identified well north of *10,000* phytochemicals and are constantly discovering new benefits from consuming these micronutrients.

Any single piece of fruit you eat is a vastly superior source of quick energy and healthy goodness than all the Gatorade you could drink in your whole life.

But, again, let's go back to the "Big Race". Elite athletes, whether amateur or professional, *are* special cases. Training for the Olympics or competing in an Iron Man Triathlon is so far outside the pale of even an average sporty existence that different rules apply.

Yet whether you're training for your first or your twentieth marathon, it's not likely you are overweight in the first place, so eating in the middle of the Glycemic Index — where there are plenty of sugars and even some low-hanging Mega-Sugars — is a perfectly viable strategy.

Whenever possible though, make fruit your carbohydrate of choice. Your beautiful body will certainly thank you for it.

The more we can wean sugars and Mega-Sugars from our lives and diets, the further down the GI scale we will go…and before long we'll find ourselves eating in the same natural fashion as all of humanity from the dawn of civilization until just a couple of brief generations ago!

And that lifestyle, ladies and gentlemen, is where the *health* lives!

"What we eat has changed more in the last forty years than in the previous forty thousand."
—Eric Schlosser

KEY #12:
"Checking Our Work"

Do Carbohydrates Really Make Us Fat?

Back in school we were often required to stop and check our work, to make sure we were doing the problems correctly, that we understood the concepts behind them clearly, and/or to determine if our answers jibed with the facts as they were being presented to us.

So now let's do a quick check our work so far, shall we? Let's test our new understanding of the actual scientific mechanism for how our bodies gain fat and lose fat against a large population—and let's call that population the United States of America.

At the heart of what we've learned so far is that while sugars are bad for us and lead to increased Insulin, increased waistlines and increased health problems, carbohydrates (or Mega-Sugars) are even *worse* for us in every category.

Whether you call them by their Big Food-approved name of carbohydrates, their more accurate chemical name of saccharides, or their gangsta street name of Mega-Sugars, my contention is that they are killing us, a pound at a time.

This is not new information…it's just information that has not been shared with us, for whatever reason. The science behind everything I've revealed to you so far has been known for years or even decades.

Now something happened in the United States back

in 1992 that will provide a perfect canvas for us to test the strengths or merits of the new eating strategy I've been laying out for you — a strategy that I contend will give you more energy, more vitality, more clarity and (last, but not least) less weight.

To understand this seminal event in 1992 that marked a dramatic turning point in the health and weight of Americans, let's travel back in time a few years *before then* in order to get the lay of the land, as they say...

1985

Thanks to the 500,000 channels now available on cable TV, there's no lack of movies, TV shows and music videos from the 1980's for us to peruse. If you haven't already done so, seriously take the time to spend an evening doing a mini-marathon of entertainment from the '80s.

What you'll be struck by again and again (and again) is how damn *thin* almost everybody seemed to be back then.

Sure, there were some overweight people, but not that many, and truly obese people were few and far between. We weren't all as skinny as the Talking Heads, but it sure seemed like it!

Here's what obesity looked like in America in 1985, thanks to the hard-working record-keepers over at the Centers for Disease Control (CDC):

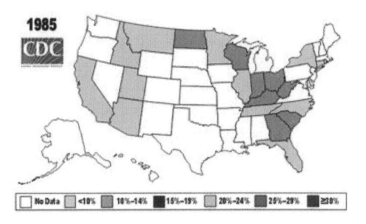

Not too shabby, especially considering that fast-food restaurants promoting a 24-hour a day carbohydrate-driven lifestyle were already starting to pop up everywhere like mushrooms on shit, as we say here in the colorful state of Texas! (If you're seeing this in glorious Black & White, as a general rule the darker the color the higher the rate of obesity in a given state. Bottom line, the only "good" color on this and following graphics is white...anything else is "non-good"!)

Sure there's a few light blue states, representing a growing incidence of obesity, and even a couple of troubling medium blue states.

But something is going on behind the scenes that should give us hope for the future. Our government is cooking up (heh-heh) a little program that should turn things around.

Over at the United States Department of Agriculture (USDA) they're already putting together what will ultimately be called the Food Pyramid. This is intended to be a handy-dandy chart of what we ought to eat and in what proportions.

The thinking behind the Food Pyramid is that since most Americans are completely unschooled in the mechanisms by which we convert glucose to fat (via Insulin) or to energy (via Glucagon) that the very least the USDA could do for us was give us a Dietary Cheat Sheet, so people could just glance at it and know what we should be eating and what we should be avoiding. Oh boy, I can't wait to see what they come up with!

1992

Let's go LIVE to 1992! It's an exciting day! The USDA is about to release their official Food Pyramid, which will take all the guess-work out of healthy eating for Americans from now on.

All we have to do is eat according to what the Food Pyramid teaches us and we'll live happily and healthily forever after.

Obesity in America can now become a thing of the past, just a little hiccup in our history.

Let's hope they get it right, since one of the principal goals of this nutritional campaign is to teach *children* a lifetime strategy of what to eat for maximum health.

So we've got no margin of error here with this new Food Pyramid thingie — our children's lives and futures are literally at stake!

But before rolling out the new Food Pyramid, let's check in with the nation's health here in 1992.

Honestly, we've gone a little downhill in the past few years...

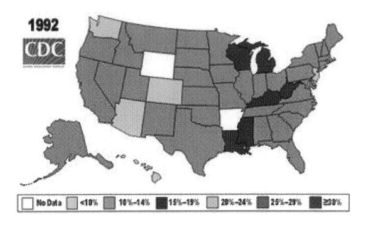

Whoa, this is not looking good. The rise and rise of the Fast-Food Nation is already taking its toll. There's already a bunch more light and medium blue states—representing 10-14% obesity rates—and we're even starting to see a couple of dark blue states, where an incredible 15% or more of the population is obese.

Hey, it's a damn good thing the US Government is about to step in with their years-in-the-making food guidelines, because, clearly, Americans are eating the wrong things and we're starting to get a little fat around here.

We definitely need some good dietary advice for a change. Without further ado, here it is, courtesy of the United States Department of Agriculture: the original Food Pyramid of 1992!

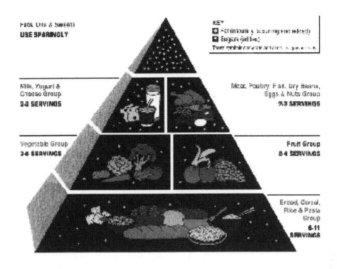

No, no, no, this can't be right! Seriously, there must be some mistake here!

An inconvenient little thing called *science* teaches us that for humans to survive we need...

Protein

Fat

Fiber

And nothing else!

Yet these 3 categories are clustered at the top of the pyramid, where we are shown and told to eat less of them *combined* than of the bottom-most "food group", which is the completely unnecessary and fattening category of carbohydrates such as breads, cereals and pastas.

In other words, the Food Pyramid is telling us to eat exactly the *opposite* of everything we've learned so far in the *Low Carb Revolution*.

I hate to admit it, since I put so much doggone work into sharing all the information in this book with you, but maybe *they* are the ones who got it right here, not me.

After all, they *are* the United States Department of Agriculture and presumably they know what the hell they're talking about, wouldn't you think?!

If they say that carbohydrates/saccharides should form the *base* of the Pyramid, and that's what we should be eating more of than anything else, who am I to say otherwise?!

Still, it seems more than a little unbelievable that their "advice" will actually work.

During the years from 1985 to the present year of 1992, we've seen that Americans have begun to fatten up from the high-carb lifestyle of the growing Fast Food Revolution.

And yet the government is encouraging us to eat even *more* carbohydrates in order to...lose weight?! I mean, every food depicted in the base of the pyramid ranks at the very *top* of the Glycemic Index.

Color me dubious, but, okay, we'll play this game!

"Eating high-carbohydrate (high-glycemic) meals three times a day and at bedtime can cause Insulin to be elevated for eighteen out of twenty-four hours. The pancreas needs a reset, and so do fat cells. Imagine Insulin pushing fat into cells eighteen hours a day!"
—Morrison Bethea, MD, Sam Andrews, MD, Leighton Stewart & Luis Balart, MD in *SUGAR BUSTERS!*

The USDA apparently begs to differ with the above scientific fact.

If a high-carb, low-fat diet IS a scientifically accurate method for Americans to return to our Ideal Weights, then I have completely wasted your time up in this book up until now...and please accept my heart-felt apologies in advance should this turn out to be the case!

If the high-carb, low-fat diet promoted by the Food Pyramid is scientifically sound, then the upward rise of obesity in America should immediately reverse itself and we should enjoy a quick return to the more "normal" statistics of the mid-eighties.

In short, if the USDA is *right*, then the unavoidable result of the Food Pyramid of 1992 *must* be a return to the obesity levels of 1985 or even lower.

Meanwhile, if what you and I have learned so far in the *Low Carb Revolution* is true, then the exact opposite of that should occur—obesity levels should not only continue to rise, but they will probably rise at a faster pace than ever before because of the dubious advice that we now fill up on the foods that make us the fattest.

Okay, let's give the Food Pyramid a good decade to show what it can do and zoom forward to the year 2002!

2002

Hi, welcome to the year 2002! Oh boy, we made it through Y2K and all the computers kept working and the world didn't end, but things are starting to get strange around here.

Everybody—and I mean *everybody*—seems to be putting on weight these days.

But maybe that's just a coincidence. So let's see how things worked out with that whole high-carb, low-fat Food Pyramid idea.

Again, if the USDA's advice was correct, if eating a diet high in Mega-Sugars really is sound nutritional advice, then the newest obesity map should show distinct and observable improvement in our obesity levels.

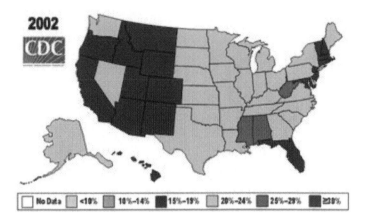

Holy Mother of Zeus, what's going on here?!

Not only has the Food Pyramid—with its "healthy" recommendation that we make carbohydrates the basis of our entire diet—*not* led to a reduction in the prevalence of obesity, the numbers of obese Americans is now off the freakin' charts!

Ten years of filling up on breads, grains, pasta and other wheat products has turned our obesity trend into a full-blow obesity *epidemic*!

We've actually got two new colors we've never even *seen* before on the latest graphic from the CDC!

(Again, the darker the color, the greater the obesity. The key at the bottom of the graphic represents low levels of obesity in the colors on the left of the scale and greater levels of obesity as the colors move to the right.)

One of the new colors on this map indicates that obesity levels have soared to over 20% in nearly half the states! You gotta be kidding me?!

Plus there are now three states where more than 25% of their fine citizens are obese!

This is a terrible, terrible turn of events.

The Low Carb Revolution by John McLean

"Advice to cut fat intake and replace the calories with whole grains coincides precisely with the start of the sharp upward climb in body weight for men and women."
—Dr. William Davis

I mean, *of course* all those carbohydrates found in bread, pasta and the now-ubiquitous mega-sweetener, High Fructose Corn Syrup, overwhelm our bloodstreams with glucose, causing abnormally high levels of Insulin, causing abnormally high levels of fat being stored and guarded and causing abnormally low levels of the appetite-suppressing hormone Leptin, so we keep eating more carbs even as we get fatter.

But adding insult to injury is the fact that this vicious high-carb cycle has the official endorsement of the United States of America.

The USDA's dietary recommendations weren't just for a High-Carb diet, but also for a Low-Fat diet. Their specific instructions about fat are: "Use Sparingly."

As the with high-carbohydrate advice, Americans listened. Following the introduction of the Food Pyramid in 1992, the percentage of fat consumed per American *decreased* by from 40 percent to the 30 percent goal targeted by the USDA.

Yet the less fat we ate, the fatter we got!

World-renowned heart surgeon Dr. Dwight Lundell aptly sums the unfolding tragedy of the faulty dietary guidelines: "We simply followed the recommended mainstream diet that is low in fat and high in carbohydrates, not knowing we were causing repeated injury to our blood vessels. This repeated injury creates chronic inflammation leading to heart disease, stroke, diabetes and obesity. Let me repeat that: The injury and inflammation in our blood vessels is *caused* by the low fat diet recommended for years by mainstream medicine."

133

So how did government officials and scientists react to the fact that Americans were actually following the recommendations of the High-Carb Pyramid and it was *causing* us grow obese at alarming rates?!

They said it was *our* fault.

They said we must still be eating too much and exercising too little, and *that* was the reason for the explosion in our weight. They said that if we would just consume fewer calories, we would magically weigh less...even though it is physically impossible to lose weight on the high-carbohydrate diet they are telling us to eat unless we are elite-level athletes like, say, Michael Phelps training for the next Olympics!

Sorry, I'm just a little steamed here. I won't go so far as saying we were lied to, but I have to wonder...

Why Were We Told to Eat The Worst Possible Foods?

Listen, I understand how the world works. The United States Department of Agriculture is *not* in the business of presiding over the health of the American populace. (Frankly, we're pretty much on our own in that area!) The USDA *is*, however, in the business of selling food. And not just to us, but to the rest of the world. Corn, soy, wheat and other high-carbohydrate food groups are major sources of export dollars for the nation.

So I get that the USDA has to advocate a high-carbohydrate diet to Americans in order for Big Food to be able to sell these same crops to other nations looking for cheap calories.

After all, if the USDA were to actually *warn* us of the health dangers of the high-carbohydrate lifestyle, then the number of overseas buyers of US crops would drop to zero.

And that would be bad...business. But it doesn't make it right.

"Those who know the least, obey the best."

—George Farquhar

The Rest of the Story

The story doesn't end there. We still have one last, up-to-date chart to consider.

But before we look at the latest map of obesity in America, let me add one final, sad note. The truth is even worse than we're being shown.

These graphics from the CDC only count the *obese* population in the United States—the fattest of the fat, with BMIs in excess of 30. They don't even include the largest percentage of the American population, those of us who are "merely" overweight.

Therefore people with near-obese BMIs of 28 or 29—and there are *millions* of us—are still classified as "overweight" rather than "obese" and so aren't even included in these graphics.

In other words, the ongoing damage to America's health from the USDA's insistence that we base our eating habits around a high-carbohydrate diet is even gloomier than the depressing picture of the nation's health and weight being graphically illustrated in these charts from the Centers for Disease Control.

"From the 1980's on we have gotten fatter and sicker. Simultaneously, our government pushed USDA foods because they realized they could make it dirt cheap and export it all over the world while making tons of money doing so."
—Jack Kruse, MD

2010

It is with a heavy heart that I present to you the most recent map of obesity levels in America...

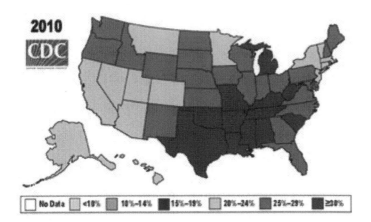

This is beyond tragic. I seriously feel like crying every time I look at this latest map. There aren't even any dark blue states left!

Even the relatively "healthy" states now have a more than 20% prevalence of obesity!

The number of medium orange states, with greater than 25% of their population categorized as obese, has exploded.

And there's even a whole new *color*, a nasty burnt orange or something, for states where more than 30% of their citizens are obese. This is freakin' crazy!

I mean, we've totally run out of colors in just twenty years of living according to the High-Carb Pyramid created by the collaboration of politicians and the Big Food corporations who fund their re-election campaigns. Next they're gonna have to invent yet *another* color as states start surpassing the 35% obesity level...as they surely will.

Whenever I look at that graphic, I think, "Wow! Just...wow!"

In merely twenty short years, this whole Eat-Carbs-to-Lose-Weight experiment has been an unmitigated disaster! It has destroyed the baseline health of an entire nation and led directly to the United States becoming not just the fattest country in the world...but also the fattest country in the *history* of the world!

As William Davis, MD, notes: "Americans are plagued by obesity on a scale never before seen in the human experience. No demographic has escaped the weight gain crisis."

After all this, you would imagine the USDA might, oh, I dunno, go back and reexamine their strategy or something?!

Maybe have a look at what *science* has known for decades about how we store fat (via Insulin) and how we lose fat (via Glucagon) and what initiates that whole process?!

The physiological mechanisms for how we actually gain weight is not difficult to understand. YOU understand it now and you could probably teach it to any government official or Big Food lackey who was willing to listen.

> *"The low-fat, more-grain message also proved enormously profitable for the processed food industry. It triggered an* explosion of *processed food products, most requiring just a few pennies worth of basic materials. Wheat flour, cornstarch, high-fructose corn syrup, sucrose and food coloring are now the main ingredients of products that fill the interior aisles of any modern supermarket."*
> — Dr. William Davis

From Obesity Crisis to Obesity Nightmare

In any case, shouldn't the USDA have one or two actual scientists or something on staff who could explain this stuff to them?! Or even a single smart guy with a white lab coat and a pocket liner and a community college education in biology?

Or just *one* person with the decency to put the American people before American business?! Because clearly something has to be done. The dietary advice we were given in the High-Carb Pyramid is so demonstrably wrong and has led us so directly into a full-blown Nightmare of Obesity that something *must* change.

Our High-Carb lifestyle isn't affecting just our weight, but also our lives.

In short, *carbohydrates are destroying our health!*

In 1900, about 650,000 Americans had diabetes. By 2010, according to the American Diabetes Association, 26 *million* children and adults in the United States suffered from diabetes, and another 80 million are afflicted with pre-diabetes.

And it's just getting worse, as an additional 2 *million* Americans (and growing) are newly diagnosed with diabetes each year.

In other words, we're now creating three times as many diabetics *each year* as there were total diabetics in the United States just a century earlier!

The reason we have become fat is not your fault or mine. It's not the fault of the average American on the street. And it's not the fault of our children. We've just been dutifully following *their* guidelines and *their* instructions.

For the past twenty years we've done what politicians, the media and Big Food has *told* us to do...which is to eat more Mega-Sugars than anything else, while limiting our consumption of real foods like fruits, vegetables, meats and fish. But maybe there's still hope.

Maybe somebody in the government will help wake us up from this national nightmare.

"Every woman knows that all carbohydrates are fattening, this is a piece of common knowledge, which few nutritionists would dispute."
—British Journal of Nutrition, 1963

The USDA Switches to "Plan B"

Indeed, in recent times a new ray of hope seemed to emerge from the USDA. Even *they* could see that Plan A clearly wasn't working out for any of us. Two decades of insisting that we consume 33% of our total daily intake of food as carbohydrates resulted in an unprecedented rise in the numbers of obese Americans...and with it, lots of negative attention about how the Food Pyramid had failed us.

Well, politicians on both sides of the aisle couldn't be seen standing around doing nothing in the face of the worst health crisis in American history, could they?!

So the politicians instructed the USDA to come up with Plan B! Upon which the "best and the brightest" at the USDA and their counterparts at the Department of Health and Human Services (HHS) went back to the drawing boards.

First they tossed out the old-fashioned High-Carb Pyramid with its ridiculous, counter-productive recommendation that we obtain fully one-third of our daily calories from carbohydrates.

Second they gathered together across boardroom tables and in front of white boards and around water coolers to determine exactly what we should eat from now on.

After several of years of intense work, meetings with lobbyists and tens of thousands of man-hours of combined effort, in 2011 the USDA came out with an all-new strategy for reversing the nationwide obesity epidemic...

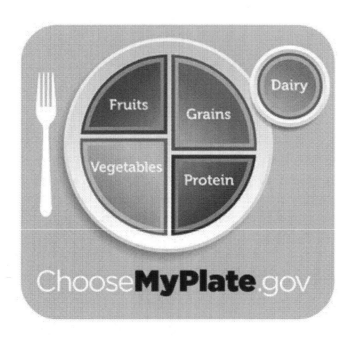

Gone are the days of making carbohydrates 33% or more of our daily intake of "food".

Instead, the new and improved plan to halt the obesity epidemic in its track and return America to mid-'80s obesity levels suggests that we lower our daily consumption of carbohydrates to...wait for it...wait for it...

...25%!

You read that right! We are now being told that "only" **25% of our daily intake of food should consist of carbohydrates!** Which, again, is just an Orwellian Newspeak term for Mega-Sugars!

These are the very same carbohydrates that occupy the top rungs of the Glycemic Index. These are the same carbohydrates that led to an unprecedented explosion in obesity and Type II Diabetes in the past twenty years. And these are the precise carbohydrates that cause our bloodstream to flood with fat-storing Insulin so we cannot help but continue to gain weight when we consume them.

There's a word for these recommendations that we maintain 25% of our diet as carbohydrates…**insane**.

It's as insane as telling a two-pack-a-day smoker that the road to restoring her health is to by all means continue smoking—but to cut back to "only" 1 ½ packs per day. Because if she stopped smoking completely, well, Big Tobacco might go out of business or something. So she should keep on smoking, but smoke just a little bit less and everybody will be happy.

Except everybody won't be happy.

> *"Just because a million people believe a lie, doesn't make it true."*
> —Buddha

It Gets Worser and Worser

Knowing what you now know about the Glycemic Index and how we create and store fat in our bodies, what do you imagine is going to happen if Americans follow this new and "improved" Food Plate where they're still being advised to consume 25% of their daily calories in the form of high-GI, high-Insulin-producing carbohydrates?!

What do you think the obesity chart is going to look a year from now or ten years from now? Will it get better? Or will it just continue to grow worse?

What are the odds that if Americans continue to eat

at the tippy top of the Glycemic Index and continue to flood their bloodstream with fat-storing Insulin that they will magically begin losing weight and the obesity epidemic will begin to recede?

Obviously, the answer is: 0%.

We are still being ordered to eat the very things that caused us to become fat in the first place.

Telling us to make "only" 25% of our total diet the things that cause us to gain weight—rather than the previous total of 33%--is pretty much the worst advice in the history of anybody ever giving anybody else advice, wouldn't you agree?!

Should you ever visit the official United States government MyPlate website, you will discover that you (and your children) are being advised to eat 5-8 portions per day from the high-carb bread and grain family of "foods"!

Reading as if it came straight from an over-the-top piece of humor writing from the satirical newspaper, *The Onion*, the offiial MyPlate website gives us examples of what the USDA and HHS are insisting we should eat 5-8 portions per day of.

The list includes nothing but fattening, top-of-the-Glycemic-Index fare such as...

Bagels
Biscuits
Breads
Pancakes
Popcorn
Breakfast cereals

Seriously?! One-quarter of the total calories we consume each day are supposed to include pancakes...popcorn...and sugary breakfast cereals?!

Again, there's really no other word to describe this dietary "advice" other than *insane!*

"I believe that the increased consumption of grains — or more accurately, the increased consumption of this genetically altered thing called modern wheat — explains the contrast between the slender, sedentary people of the fifties and overweight twenty-first century people, triathletes included."
— William Davis, MD

Time for "Plan U"

Suppose you had a teenage daughter, and you found out she was drinking a 6-pack of beer each day.

Would you say to her, "Oh, honey, drinking so much alcohol will stunt your growth and cause all sorts of health problems. Don't drink a 6-pack of beer each day. Instead, just drink 4 beers. I mean the beer companies have to sell beer, so I'm not going to say drink no beers, because that would hurt their profits and then how would politicians afford to get re-elected, but I just want you to drink a little more moderately and get a little less drunk and then everybody will be happy"?!

Except, once more, everybody *won't* be happy.

For 20 years now a High-Carb diet has enjoyed the full support of politicians on both sides of the aisle who depend on $$$ from Big Food's army of well-heeled lobbyists to further their political careers.

I'd like to suggest that these politicians no longer deserve a say in how you live your life and treat your body.

They have bungled away the opportunity to give you or me or any human alive any dietary advice whatsoever. They have permanently forfeited away the right to tell us what to eat or not eat based on their deplorable track record with the trusting people of the

United States who followed them down this dark alley of excess sugars and carbohydrates.

First we had the High-Carb Pyramid. Now we have the High-Carb Plate.

I view the two of these as sort of the *Exxon Valdez* and *Costa Concordia* of the nutrition world...object lessons in how *not* to live unless our specific goal is failure.

In terms of *your* weight and *your* health, all that matters is that you are happy!

Ultimately, the only person who gets to decide what you eat and how much you eat is YOU!

So it's time for "Plan U" — as in "You"!

Now that we've checked our work and seem to be on the right track together, let's keep learning more about what you can personally do to create some magnificent changes in your life, shall we?!

> *"Ultimately the only power to which man should aspire is that which he exercises over himself."*
> — Elie Wiesel

Reality Check

Before we jump into the next bit of awesomeness, let's do a final Reality Check here.

In truth, most Americans do *not* follow the MyPlate orders that we take in 25% of our total daily input of food and drink in the form of carbohydrates. We do not even consume the original High-Carb Pyramid's commandment that 33% of our total daily intake must be carbs.

It turns out that Americans consume approximately **55%** of their total daily calories in the form of carbohydrates!

More than half of our total daily calories comes from

Insulin-spiking, fat-storing carbohydrates. And that is the sole reason behind our growing Obesity Nightmare. Period.

In the chapters ahead I'm going to encourage you and nudge you in the direction of a lifestyle where you'll eat fewer carbohydrates than you may be accustomed to.

I naturally don't expect you to ever get all the way to 0% carbs and stay there forever. The goal here is for every step—every progression, as I term it—to be both enjoyable and sustainable.

If you number among the people who now consume half or more of their daily calories in the form of carbohydrates/saccharides, then cutting back to 33% or even 25% would reap enormous benefits in your health and waistline.

As you eat fewer carbs, you'll feel better, you'll have more energy and more vitality, more clarity in your thinking and your love life will improve beyond your wildest dreams. (I mean, why not?! I doubt there's any scientific studies proving that lower carbs leads to a better love life, but there's also probably no scientific proof that this isn't true, either!)

The takeaway here: do what you can to lower your carbs, and love yourself for every positive step you take on this wonderful journey.

Hey, kids, here's a final idea for us to consider:

What do you say we air-drop a bunch of copies of Dr. Spock's classic baby book on the USDA and the Department of Health & Human Services so they, too, can discover the "Breaking News of 1946" that starches and other carbohydrates alone determine how much weight we gain!

The Low Carb Revolution by John McLean

"The amount of plain, starchy foods (cereals, breads, potatoes) taken in is what determines, in most people, how much weight they gain or lose."
— Dr. Spock's Baby and Child Care, six editions, 1946-1992

(You might be painfully bemused to note the passages about carbohydrates in starchy foods and grains causing weight gain were mysteriously and permanently EXPUNGED from the text of Dr. Spock's classic work following the USDA's released their High-Carb Pyramid in 1992! No subsequent editions mention this formerly well-known fact.)

KEY #13:
"Gearing Up for the Low Carb Revolution"

Welcome to the Best Health of Your Life!

Ready for some good news? We've now made it through all the science-y bits of the book and have built an incredible foundation for the transformational work we're going to do together from here on out.

For the rest of Part One we're going to move from the general to the specific. We've learned how our bodies work from the inside-out.

Now it's time to learn how to apply that knowledge so we can change our bodies from the outside-in...through the food and drink we put into it.

In this chapter, we'll get a road map for the next leg of our amazing journey together.

This map includes an overview of the 13 Progressions that form the beating heart of the *Low Carb Revolution* lifestyle. As you incorporate each of these progressions into your life, you'll increasingly notice some amazing benefits for yourself.

Lose Weight
Gain Energy
More Vitality
Greater Clarity

Let's briefly explore each of these *benefits* in turn.

Benefit #1: Lose Weight

Losing weight is the first and most obvious benefit of the *Low Carb Revolution* lifestyle, to be sure. You are now thoroughly versed in the science of how our

147

bodies store fat from a high-carb/high-Insulin lifestyle...and you also now understand how to trigger the fat-burning response from the hormone Glucagon by *avoiding* carbohydrates and incorporating lower Glycemic Index eating into your life. (This also means you are now officially unemployable at the United States Department of Agriculture, lulz!)

Mind you, we'll learn the *details* of exactly how to eat low GI in the chapters ahead, as well as additional strategies and techniques to accelerate the pace of the transformations we're undergoing.

As encouraging and empowering as it is to step on the scale each day and watch the numbers dwindle, I personally believe that losing weight itself will eventually become one of the least interesting benefits to you in this entire process.

Sure, you'll lose weight...but perhaps even more important to your future and your happiness is what you'll be *gaining*!

Benefit #2: Gain Energy

When you really live this lifestyle, you'll have energy to burn...literally!

You'll meet your energy needs primarily through the two food groups that are required to sustain life: protein and fat. Protein can stimulate Insulin — but only mildly and not in high enough quantities to cause any negative effects on our waistline.

On the other hand, Insulin and fat are not even on speaking terms.

Insulin completely ignores fat, which allows it to be used in abundance for our daily energy needs.

And by fat I mean the natural fats that make up avocados and nuts and eggs and coconut oil and animal products from fish to beef to chicken and everything in between.

Most people experience a surge in their energy levels as they advance through the 13 Progressions that make up this lifestyle.

Each new distinction gives them even more access to the amazing power of their own body. I personally have so much available energy from my *Low Carb Revolution* lifestyle that I sometimes play for up to 4 hours per day (or even more, when I attend week- or weekend-long dance workshops and retreats, as I often do) without growing tired in the least.

For me, "play" means a daily walk or bicycle ride of about an hour. It includes almost daily dancing, as well as time spent swimming, juggling, climbing trees and horsing around with my children. I have unlimited amounts of energy to do any physical activity I desire without ever needing to take in added carbohydrates or "Energy" bars or "Sports" drinks or any of the other fattening liquidious concoctions marketed deliberately to turn active people into inactive, television-watching, internet-shopping meat robots.

And my super-high energy levels have nothing to do with age, since I'm old enough to have a 21 year-old daughter, an 18 year-old son and a 13 year-old half-daughter (long story)! My children variously put my age at just over a century all the way up to fully 2000 years...so if I can do it, so can you!

As you embrace the *Low Carb Revolution* lifestyle, your body will transition from being dependent on the immediate energy of carbohydrates to learning how to create energy from your own fat stores in a super-awesome process called *gluconeogenesis*.

Gluco-Neo-Something-or-Another

This is an important concept to understand, so let's briefly break down this process called gluconeogenesis...

Gluco — as in glucose, the fuel that all life forms use to power their engines

Neo — as in brand new...and coincidentally the name of the lead character in the seminal movie about "waking up", *The Matrix*

Genesis — the process of being born and/or one of the greatest English rock bands of all time

So *gluconeogenesis* means "giving birth to new glucose".

And where does our body get the raw materials to create new glucose which we can convert to energy?

From our stored *fat*, that's where, baby!

And the more we rely on this process of burning our own fat for our energy needs — rather than depending on added carbs — the more *sustainable* our energy expenditures will be.

Here's how I think about it...carbohydrates are like the lighter fluid of the food world. Sure, lighter fluid flames up instantly, but it also burns itself out quickly. You have to keep adding more and more lighter fluid to keep a tiny fire burning in the barbeque grill, but it's never gonna burn hot enough or long enough to cook anything on its own.

A better strategy for building a barbeque, of course, is to use wood or coal as your fire source. It takes a little longer to get going, no doubt, but it burns longer and is infinitely sustainable so long as you keep adding fuel in the form of additional wood or coal.

Once you have a fire burning inside you that doesn't depend on lighter fluid (carbohydrates), your fire will just keep burning and burning and burning so long as you occasionally add fuel (protein and fat, tempered with a measure of fiber to make sure you're pooping plenty!) — you will never run out of energy either!

When you reach that point, lemme know, because then we'll go out dancing together, you and I, and we'll just keep dancing and dancing the entire night, while all the people around us who depend on "lighter fluid" for their fuel have to stop every 4-5 songs to go get more lighter fluid in the form of an alcoholic drink or pretzels or something so they have the energy to dance another four or five songs until they have to refuel yet again—and then we'll win the big dance competition and get our pictures in the newspaper and probably even win a little trophy!

And all thanks to gluconeogenesis!

Benefit #3: More Vitality

If you recall, I characterize Energy as the power to move our bodies through space, while Vitality is the "inner energy" it takes to sit still and create.

Any fool can muster the energy to dash from Point A to Point B. And any fool can sit around and enjoy the creations of others by watching TV or reading a magazine.

However, no fool is able to sit down and create original work of their own. When fools *do* sit down to create, they quickly realize their internal battery is completely drained and they simply don't have the "vitality" to keep their butts in the seat and get anything done.

If you are ever going to write the Great American Novel (and I sincerely hope you do!) you're going to require a great deal of vitality to sit down, day after day for some months or more in order to write your book!

One of the great, unexpected benefits of the revolutionary new lifestyle you're now embracing is the increased vitality it will bring to you and your creative and/or wealth-building projects.

Just to give you an idea of the vitality (or inner energy) I am able to tap into living my low-carbohydrate lifestyle, I wrote the *Low Carb Revolution* from scratch in just 47 days.

We're talking about a book of 464 pages with some 115,000 words in just under seven weeks, from start to finish. And I didn't have an outline or so much as a single sheet of notes on the day I started! And this certainly isn't because I'm some kind of freakish workaholic.

Far from it — if anything, I'm a *Playaholic*!

I rarely wrote for more than 4-5 hours per day during those 47 days, but I had so much vitality at my disposal because of the fire burning in my core that every moment I spent writing translated almost directly into goodness on the page.

While we're on the subject, if you are enjoying my book, please tell other members of your Tribe about it so they'll have same opportunity as you to reconnect with their beautiful bodies and go on this amazing journey of self-discovery.

If you feel the *Low Carb Revolution* deserves a 5-Star review, then pay a quick visit to Amazon.com and share your feelings with the rest of the class. I look forward to reading your comments!

And if you've finally ready to sit down and write your own book — you know, the one that's been percolating within you for half a lifetime — then head on over to Amazon and check out my 220-page book on the subject, GET PUBLISHED NOW! The Step-by-Step Guide to Writing & Publishing Your First Book on Amazon Kindle!

As you begin adopting the progressions that follow, you will find yourself able to tap into greater and greater vitality in your life.

And as you do, I would love for you to put that vitality to use. I would love for you to create more. I mean, what's the point of doing all of this — of letting go of the old weight and totally transforming our lives—if we're not going to use the experience to open ourselves up to *create* more?!

And by "creating" I don't just mean creating art, far from it. I mean creating art and creating wealth and creating happiness in our life and the lives of those around us...and creating more love and forgiveness and creating a better world. I think you get the idea!

Benefit #4: Greater Clarity

We will build and expand upon your newfound clarity throughout the *Low Carb Revolution*. As we begin to handle our bodies and love our bodies and love ourselves, opportunities will arise for us to really wake up and finally "get here".

The clarity that naturally emerges during this process is one of the most powerful benefits we can experience. Because the more clarity we have, the closer we come to "waking up" from the slumbers we've been in our entire lives.

And Waking Up, ultimately, is the point of this *entire* journey.

For some, it's a slow, gradual, measured awakening to the possibilities of life. For others, it manifests in an instant—a signal moment in our lives where we arise one morning, look down at ourselves and realize we have become someone different than who we were for the first kazillion years of being us.

Whether slow or fast, Waking Up leads to a momentous realization and understanding of Who We Are and Why We Are Here.

Not only is that one of the most beautiful experiences possible, but it's also your eventual destination if you continue reading all the way through to the end of the *Low Carb Revolution* and keep applying the strategies and learnings into your life.

When you arrive at that point and you later pass up

reaching for a high-carb "food" to eat, you may not even think deliberately about the fat that would be stored in your cells because of it...instead you'll realize *it was the carbohydrates that put you to sleep in the first place and that the secret to staying awake is to simply eat fewer of them!*

What Are "Progressions"?

Something you may or may not know about me is that I'm a juggler! Not only do I juggle, but I also teach other people to juggle. In fact, I can even teach YOU how to juggle!

The best way to teach juggling — or anything, for that matter — is to break down whatever your teaching into the smallest possible units, which I refer to as *progressions*, and then teach these one at a time.

If you ever learn to juggle, you'll start with a 1st Progression of a single ball, which you'll learn to throw from one hand to the other and then back again.

Only once you've mastered throwing that one ball from hand to hand do we move on to the 2nd Progression, which is — you guessed it — throwing two balls. And so on, through the five progressions in total that it takes to learn to juggle.

Likewise, all of the information in the remainder of Part One is arranged in Progressions. Only when you've mastered (whatever "mastered" means to you) one progression should you begin incorporating the next progression into your life.

In other words, read and absorb a progression...and then go off and do that thing for a day or a week or a month. And when you're ready, come back and do the next progression, and so on.

Go At Your Own Pace

I deliberately ranked the following 13 Progressions in order of importance for both losing weight and for the practically of making these changes in our eating habits and lifestyle.

The first few progressions are by far the most important. Even if you only do the first two or three or so, you will *still* put yourself in an excellent position to succeed at losing weight...and gaining many of the other benefits of a lower-carb lifestyle.

Later, as you add additional progressions, you'll continue to lose weight, as well as gain energy, experience more vitality and enjoy greater clarity than ever before.

You'll be waking up to your true power and potential! The actual timeline of implementing the following progressions is a personal choice you'll make for yourself.

My only recommendation about these progression is that you NOT attempt to do them all at once. That's just a lot—too much, really—of change to throw at your life and your body in one fell swoop.

Trying to modify too many things about ourselves or our lifestyle all at once can be a recipe for disaster. Slow, steady progress is the key to success in making lasting transformation in our life.

Take a few days or even a few weeks to implement each progression and get a lasting feel for it in your body.

Then, working hand in hand with the amazing techniques of changing your *habits* that you'll discover in Part Two, you'll be able to make each progression into a new habit in a ridiculously short amount of time.

This is doubly (or maybe even trebly!) true if you play the Audio Affirmations I've created for you in the background as you go about your day.

These affirmations were designed to support you and integrate everything we've been discovering together down to a cellular level in your body. Once again, here's the link where you listen to and/or permanently download the affirmations:

http://db.tt/69WOj7pW

Or at this alternate download site:

http://www15.zippyshare.com/v/36838740/file.html

(Simply type either of the URLs into your browser.)

Avoid vs. Eliminate

As a former 5-pack a day chain-smoker, I don't like anybody telling me I absolutely can never do something ever again. It just sorta rubs me the wrong way, and you might feel the same way.

Sometimes when people give us dietary suggestions, they go well beyond the category of suggestion and insist that we adhere to their iron-clad rule to always eat left-handed...or never eat left-handed or whatever their thing is. Sometimes we are ordered to completely eliminate certain foods or food groups from our diets, which means we can never, ever, ever have them again.

Well, we're not going to do that here! I strongly believe that when we eliminate someone's options entirely we almost deliberately set them up for failure.

Instead, I'm going to recommend you just *avoid* certain somethings. And that's a totally different thing!

By "avoid" I mean that you should mostly stay away from whatever it is if your goal is to lose weight, gain energy, wake up, etc. That doesn't mean cut it out of your life entirely, but rather avoid excess amounts of it.

For all practical purposes, you may end up avoiding some of these categories entirely for the rest of your life…but we're not even going to think about it in those terms.

For example, the second progression suggests that we Avoid Excess Sugars. That doesn't mean we may never eat dessert again ever for the rest of our lives ever! It means: eat *less* dessert-like substances than maybe we once were in the habit of eating if our goal is to "call" less Insulin into our bloodstream and thereby store less belly fat.

Because for sure, the more we avoid excess sugars such as desserts, the better we will feel, the less we'll weigh, the more awake we'll become, and on and on.

And we may end up avoiding excess sugars so much that we *do* effectively eliminate them from our diet entirely, but let's just play it by ear and see where we end up.

In a sense you could say that I'm not going to insist that you break up with "beans" entirely…instead just play really, really hard to get!

"The secret to staying young is to live
honestly, eat slowly and lie about your age."
—Lucille Ball

The 13 Progressions of the Low Carb Revolution

1) Eat as much as you want

2) Avoid Excess Sugars

3) Avoid Wheat Products

4) Drink Alcohol in Moderation

5) Avoid Processed Carbs

6) Avoid Drinking Sugars & Carbs

7) Avoid Natural Carbs

8) Mind your pH

9) Mix It Up

10) Cook It Yourself

11) Love

12) Create

13) Wake Up

PROGRESSION #1:
Eat as Much as You Want

Christine's Cat

Some years ago I dated a criminal defense attorney named Christine. And Christine owned a cat. An ancient, fluffy, jet-black cat...one of those well-fed apartment cats that have grown too old to venture out into the big bad world full of dogs and serial killers and whatever else they have out there.

Getting into and out of Christine's apartment was always a major production because her cat spent every waking moment trying to figure out how to escape.

The cat would stare at the door for endless hours trying to come up with plans for getting outside. He would pace the living room, calculating what possible trajectory and speed and angle might allow him to finally break free. Every time you opened or closed the apartment door, the stir-crazy cat would make some sort of attempt to jump, squeeze, run or claw his way outside. But the cat never made it, and never would, because Christine just knew he would be killed by a dog or car or falling meteorite or something if he so much as set a single paw out of doors.

One evening, Christine went to bed early. It was just me and the cat and the most recent summer Olympics on TV.

Now this was back when I still smoked cigarettes. Later on I'll tell the story of what a furious, nearly five-pack-a-day (egads!) chain-smoker I used to be. Suffice it say that back then I could barely sit through even the 100-meter dash without a cigarette. Or perhaps two cigarettes, what with replays and all!

So that evening, while my then-girlfriend was asleep, I decided I was going to just smoke in the living room of her apartment while I watched the Olympics. To that end, I set up a fan and then opened the door to blow the cigarette smoke out.

Upon which Christine's cat shot out the door faster than world-record holder Usain Bolt. As I knew it would.

But I also had a method to my madness...I had a plan. I sat there on the couch sipping my little vodka and chain-smoking my little cigarettes and watching the summer Olympics. "Woo-hoo, Michael Phelps wins another gold. Go Team USA!"

After about 20 minutes, Christine's cat snuck into view outside the still-open front door.

When I looked at him, the cat gave a start and bolted away. Maybe 10 minutes later, the cat walked by from the other direction, looked long and hard into the apartment, and then kept walking.

Long story short, some 45 minutes since the apartment door was originally opened and Christine's cat could finally make its long-planned escape, the cat sat purringly on the armrest of the couch right next to me, gazing idly at the open door while I scratched the top of his fuzzy head.

Christine's cat didn't particularly want to go outside.

He just wanted *to be able to go outside* if he chose.

Like we *all* do.

The All-You-Can-Eat Buffet is Now Open

Most of us have no inclination to touch a freshly painted wall while the paint is still wet.

Until…some fool puts up a sign saying: "Wet Paint--Do Not Touch!" Suddenly the desire to touch the paint wells up in us and becomes an obsession.

Must…Touch…Wet…Paint!

Even before we start making any changes in what we're eating, before we begin setting aside the "beans" — the food groups we're going to eat less of--I want you to wrap your mind around the concept that the apartment door leading to the pantry of the world is now *open.*

You can come and go anytime you like. When you are hungry, eat. When you are no longer hungry, stop eating.

Eat whatever amount you desire, without any consideration to the number of calories or the size of the portion.

Because it's not about the calories. It never was about the calories and it never will be about the calories. This you already know to the depth of your being.

Opening the door that leads to *not* counting calories and *not* measuring portions can feel so liberating, so utterly freeing. Simply giving ourselves permission to satisfy our natural hunger cravings is an important step on the road to reclaiming our birthright of our Ideal Body.

Feeling Less Hunger

In the chapters ahead we are going to explore a series of progressions that will give us the opportunity to settle into a new lifestyle at our own pace.

As we implement each progression, profound changes will be taking place deep within us. Our dutiful servant, the overworked, fat-storing hormone Insulin will get a well-deserved vacation.

Our new BFF Glucagon will gain more chances to

share its fat-releasing message with our body.

And our long-lost chum Leptin will start showing up more frequently, popping in like a Dr. Bombay returning from his travels, and telling our brains to shut down our appetite because we feel full.

One of the most delightful side effects of the *Low Carb Revolution* lifestyle is that we will naturally begin to feel less hungry as we go along. As we eat lower and lower on the Glycemic Index, we will simply feel fuller more often. Recall that Leptin, the hormone responsible for letting us know when we're no longer hungry, is blocked by the presence of Insulin within our blood supply. And the reverse is also true…

Less Insulin = more Leptin.

More and more often we'll enjoy what's referred to as *satiety*, where we feel completely content with the amount of food in our bellies and have no hunger pangs of any kind to distract us from getting on with the business of being Amazing!

Low-Carb is More Affordable

Because the food we'll be eating is so dense in nutrients and energy, we won't need as much of it as we did when we were subsisting primarily on Krap from the local McTacoHut.

Remember, the High-Carb Food Pyramid was designed by lobbyists and "nutritionists" for one reason only: to help Big Food make more money with the lowest possible cost of goods.

Despite having the lowest of all cost of goods, food-shaped chemicals made from wheat, corn, soy and sugars often cost more than actual food grown in the actual ground.

My local supermarket sells delicious rack of lamb for about $2.25 per lb. The other day I spent $3.99 for just under 2 pounds of lamb chops, which I roasted in the oven @ 325° for a few hours. When it was done, I sprinkled the lamb liberally with uncooked cilantro and parsley, then ate like a king.

For that same $3.99 I could have instead bought a big bag of Cheetos—which would've provided no nutrients, no lasting energy and a whole lot of Insulin-created fat in my body...as well as hours of orange-dyed fingertips resistant to all the soap and water in the world!

Real foods that are grown in the ground (fruits and vegetables) or on the ground (animals) are not only often cheaper than a high-carb diet, they are far more filling.

My private clients end up naturally eating less than they were accustomed to and still feeling a greater satiety from each meal.

Despite my extremely high daily energy output—again, I am sometimes physically active for 4 or more hours per day, and almost never for less than an hour or two—I sometime eat only a single sit-down meal per day, and supplement that with a combination of fruits, seeds and nuts. I regularly try to eat two sit-down meals per day, but if I'm not hungry enough for a whole second meal I don't force it on myself.

My only measure of success is: Do I have enough energy to do everything I want to do and still have energy left over at the end of the day for anything else that might come up?! If the answer to this question is "yes"—and it always is--then nothing else matters.

Counting sheep is a more effective strategy for letting go of excess pounds than counting calories! I can't repeat this often enough...

Losing weight isn't about restricting calories...it's about avoiding sugars and Mega-Sugars.

A daily, stand-up breakfast of as much fruit or

yogurt or tuna fish as I desire, followed by one or two sit-down meals with no limits to the amounts of anything I eat, provide me with all the energy—and, just as importantly, all the vitality—to easily accomplish everything I want each day.

Even so, I have no hard and fast rules of how many or how few meals I eat each day, other than giving myself going permission to eat as much as I want.

Which begs the question, *"Eat as much as I want of what?!"*

Well I'm so glad you asked! To answer, let's return to our Glycemic Index formula from earlier...

Eat High GI to GAIN a LOT of WEIGHT— **Carbohydrates & Starches (Mega-Sugars)**

Eat Mid GI to GAIN a MEDIUM AMOUNT of WEIGHT—**Sugars**

Eat Low GI to LOSE WEIGHT—**Food (Animals, Plants, Seeds & Nuts)**

Let's take a few moments to explore each strategy of eating High, Medium or Low on the Glycemic Index in turn.

Eat High GI to Gain a Lot of Weight

The Glycemic Index is a measure of the effects of carbohydrates on our blood sugar levels. Foods high in carbohydrates/saccharides spike our Insulin and cause us to gain excess weight.

So the best way to pack on the pounds is to consume as many sugars and carbohydrates as possible.

In other words, to live according to the dictates of the High-Carb Pyramid...which led Americans straight into our Obesity Nightmare in the first place!

As we'll discover in an upcoming progression, Wheat Products—including breads, pasta, cereals and the like—contain *more* carbohydrates and score higher on the Glycemic Index than every other food-like substance in existence save for pure starches.

None of the *3 essential human foods* cause us to gain weight.

Protein doesn't trigger the fat-storing Insulin response in our bloodstream unless eaten in excessive amounts.

Fat doesn't ever trigger the fat-storing Insulin response in our bloodstream.

Fiber triggers an acceptably low Insulin response in our bloodstream.

Only nutritionally unnecessary substances like simple sugars (table sugar and most sweets) and complex sugars (carbohydrates and starches) cause us to gain excess weight.

It's important to note that right now, at this juncture in our very First Progression, I am still not asking you to restrict your intake of High GI/High Carb foods.

In fact, I'm not yet asking you to avoid any "beans" at all. Yet.

All we're doing now is making ourselves *aware* of what's to come and beginning to wrap our minds around the concept of eating without the unnatural restrictions which have been placed on us all our lives. There are just two easy "homework" assignments in this progression.

The first is to let go of the counterproductive habit of counting calories. Let's give ourselves permission to eat as much as we desire whenever we desire. And the second is to pay more attention to the carbohydrates in the foods we eat.

Recall that the Glycemic Index is simply a measure of the effects of carbohydrates on our blood sugar levels.

The higher the GI of a food, the more glucose it produces, the more Insulin gets called and the more fat

165

gets stored. We've seen a list with a few samplings of high-GI foods and we'll revisit the upper end of the chart before long.

For now, though, we're just becoming more aware of the carbohydrates/GI count of the foods we are currently in the habit of eating. That's easy enough, right?!

Eat Mid-GI to Gain a Medium Amount of Weight

The next rung of the Glycemic Index ladder is different from the top only in kind. The middle of the GI is comprised largely of sugars (such as table sugar itself) and various "simple" sweets and snacks such ice cream, potato chips, candy bars, soda and wheat-free candies.

(Because Mega-Sugars like bread, pasta and rice have more carbohydrates than simple sugars like candy and ice cream, they score far higher on the Glycemic Index and are much worse for our blood sugar and waistline than "sweets". Most Americans would be better off skipping the entrée at the Olive Garden and just going straight to dessert!)

We will *still* gain weight by eating in the middle of the GI, but we'll gain less than we would living on a diet higher in carbohydrates.

If our specific goal is to lose weight, we would naturally want to avoid even the middle, sugary rungs of the Glycemic Index whenever possible and stick with the actual food of a low GI lifestyle, which doesn't cause excess blood sugar levels or weight gain.

Then, as we make good progress in returning to our Ideal Weight, occasional forays into Ice Cream Land and Candy Cane Village would be perfectly acceptable. Recall that for the greater part of human history (2 million years minus a few centuries), most humans had no access to any of the sweet substances found today in the middle of the Glycemic Index.

But you'd better believe that if they had stumbled upon a beehive or an abandoned delivery truck filled with Twinkies they would've eaten the hell out of 'em!

Eat Low GI to Lose Weight

Welcome to the area of the Glycemic Index where the food lives!

When we are actively looking to shed weight and get rid of belly fat, eating Low GI is the only way to fly, baby! The numbers separating the traditional categories of the Glycemic Index are, shall we say, quite generous.

70-100 is High
55-70 is Medium
54 & under is Low

Most actual foods—which is ultimately what we're going to strive to eat—score 35 or under, and I would recommend you eat in that range if your goal is to seriously cultivate a relationship with Glucagon and burn more stored fat on a continuous basis.

And, of course, the closer we get to 0 on the GI, the better our prospects for maintaining an exceedingly dull, boring, normal blood sugar—which is exactly what we want!

A quiet evening of normal blood sugar may look a bit dull—but it sure feels exciting on the inside!

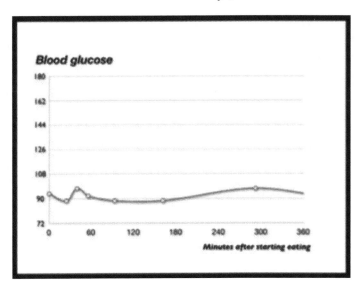

Here are the general categories of foods available for us to eat in unlimited quantities (for now...we'll cover a few minor exceptions in later progressions) as part of the *Low Carb Revolution* lifestyle.

ALL fruits – average GI of 5-30
ALL vegetables – average GI of 10-40
ALL beans – average GI of 20-40
ALL dairy (including milk, cheese, butter, etc.) – average GI of 15-45
ALL seeds & nuts – average GI of 5-25

Sort of like the game of Limbo, the lower you go, the better for your waistline! Now let's turn our attention to foods that grow on the ground or in the air or under the waves...animal foods.

Beef – GI = 0
Pork – GI = 0
Lamb – GI = 0
Fish – GI = 0
Chicken – GI = 0
Buffalo – GI = 0

Goat – GI = 0
Turkey – GI = 0
Duck – GI = 0
Any other Animal Product not listed – GI = 0

As you can see, all meat, all fish and all poultry contain zero carbohydrates and therefore score zero on the Glycemic Index. Pretty cool, huh?!

However (and this is a super-duper important "however"), remember that the three essential substances for human life are protein & fat (both found in just exactly the right proportions in the animal products described above) AND a daily dose of fiber, which is not contained in any animal products.

Since the dawn of humanity we've obtained our energy, vitamin and mineral needs from a combination of animal *and* plant foods.

That means you do not want to create a diet of 100% animal products all the time just to stay at the bottom of the Glycemic Index for maximum weight loss.

We need the nutrients, minerals and phytochemicals of vegetables and fruits to flourish AND we require the fiber in beans, seeds and plant-foods to survive.

Quick Tip: Hands down the best source of fiber is not from sugary, high-carb bread products (as Big Food/Big Diet would have us believe), but rather from all the many spectacular varieties of beans! Indeed, it's the indigestible fiber within beans that causes the notorious gases associated with them. As Anti-Sugar crusader Dr. Robert Lustig puts it, "You gotta pick one…either fat or fart!"

Progression #1: Eat as Much as You Want
YOUR NEXT STEP...

Do NOT count calories or measure portions of your food

Do NOT restrict your food choices according to High, Mid or Low GI just yet

DO eat when hungry and stop when no longer hungry

DO begin *noticing* the carbohydrates in the foods you eat

DO Google a couple of free, online sources of the Glycemic Index and start paying attention to which foods you currently eat score High, which score Mid and which score Low

> *"Food is like sex: when you abstain, even the*
> *worst stuff begins to look good!"*
> — Beth McCollister

PROGRESSION #2:
Avoid Excess Sugars

The Moment of Truth

It's time to draw a line in the sand and make a stand for our beautiful bodies. We now know what to do, and we're going to start doing it...one bold, courageous step at a time as we work our way through all 13 Progressions of the *Low Carb Revolution*.

If you are currently overweight and have a desire to return to your natural state and birthright of your Ideal Body, then you're going to have to make some fairly dramatic changes in your lifestyle. You already know that. This isn't a surprise to you or anything. You knew this moment was coming. You knew that sooner or later it was gonna be time to face facts and take action.

The High-Carb Pyramid diet—approved by politicians who depend on Big Food's lobbyists for re-election $$$—brought us to where we are today.

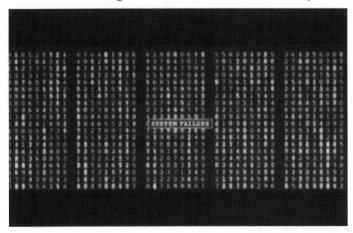

These are the same people who continue to peddle their patently false Calorie Myth of Weight Loss model to anyone and everyone who will listen. You and I know that Insulin causes fat storage and fat maintenance, not calories.

And what "causes" Insulin? Well, for starters, sugar.

Less Sugar = Less Insulin = Less Fat

In this progression we're going to kick start the beautiful transition in our bodies to a bloodstream that contains less and less of the fat-storing hormone Insulin. To accomplish this we're going to avoid excess sugars.

If you have a long, deeply ingrained habit of indulging in sweets, this vital step in the journey towards waking up to your true potential might seem difficult to even contemplate.

However, keep in mind that the entire second half of the *Low Carb Revolution* will teach you an entirely new model of how your habits are formed and how to change them. In the chapters to come, I'll take you by the hand and help you discover how to make overwhelming personal transformations in your mind, your body and your life.

In the opening 13 Keys of this book, we discovered WHY we need to make certain changes in our eating habits in order to lose weight.

In the current 13 Progressions, we'll learn exactly WHAT changes are necessary to achieve that goal.

And in the 13 Secrets that close out the book, we will explore HOW to make those changes — or any other changes we desire in our habits and lifestyle!

Avoid Excess Sugars

It's time to start limiting the excess sugars we put into our bloodstream. We're not doing this because cotton candy, M&Ms, ice cream, maple syrup and the like aren't yum-tastic. And we're not doing it because of the "calories" in these substances. We're doing it entirely to reduce the level of circulating Insulin inside ourselves. In order to lower the amount of Insulin our blood supply "calls", we must first control and limit our intake of sugars.

> *"Remember, it is not so much the ingested fat that makes you obese as the ingested sugars and carbohydrates that are converted through the influence of Insulin to fat."*
> --Morrison Bethea, MD, Sam Andrews, MD, Leighton Steward & Luis Balart, MD in *SUGAR BUSTERS!*

The more sugar we consume, the more our already over-taxed pancreas has to keep pumping out additional Insulin to keep up with the attendant glucose.

Consider this: the founders of the United States of America likely didn't secrete as much Insulin during their entire lifetime as Americans now secrete each *month* on our modern sugary diet!

We may think of ancient Rome as a time of gluttony and debauchery, but since refined sugar and manufactured carbohydrates were still more than a thousand years in their future, they were quite healthy compared to us.

Even the prominent second-century Roman physician Galen remarked that he'd only seen two cases of diabetes in all the years of his long and storied medical practice.

Fat Doesn't Cause Fat

We've already discovered that the best (indeed, only) indication of how much fat-causing Insulin we will secrete following the consumption of any food is the

173

number of sugars and carbohydrates (Mega-Sugars) it contains.

Other than dairy and eggs—which are tolerably low on the Glycemic Index and can be eaten without reservation or hesitation—all animal products made from actual animals have 0 carbohydrates and score a 0 on the GI.

Which means they do not summon Insulin and therefore when they're broken down into glucose in our bloodstreams they're burned as energy rather than stored as fat.

I regularly eat "fatty" meats such as lamb, duck, pork belly (uncured bacon) and fish—and yet I remain super-fit and super-trim and super-immodest about the whole thing! I'm 6'3" tall and weigh 189 lbs.--which is exactly what I weighed as a 17 year-old senior in high school. And I'm well-removed from my youth, with two children past high school age and another one approcahing high school any second now!

And I'm not talking about just eating "fatty types of meats", but about eating the actual fat of these fatty meats.

Don't avoid animal fat, it's the densest source of potential energy we can possibly consume!

Fat has been demonized by the Powers-That-Be (the very same ones who gave us the dietary advice that led to our ongoing Obesity Epidemic, don't ya know?!) as part of their misleading, pro-carb campaign.

Here's the calorie count for the four substances humans can eat or drink as fuel.

Protein—*4 calories per gram*
Carbohydrates—*4 calories per gram*
Alcohol—*7 calories per gram*
Fat—*9 calories per gram*

You'll notice that fat contains the most calories of all.

174

And that's the whole POINT of them! The calories I get from eating fat are what gives me the energy to run and jump and play and dance for up to 4 hours a day and still have the vitality to sit down and write books and create videos and build my business!

Animal fats and vegetable fats (such as the natural fats in cheese, dairy, avocados, seeds, nuts, etc.) are the *fuel* that fires the Low Carb Revolution lifestyle.

These necessary fats are our wood, they are our coal, they are what keeps our furnace burning red-hot day and night without needing to add the "lighter fluid of carbohydrates" to the mix.

The extra calories in animal and vegetable fats mean we naturally want to eat less of them and we naturally feel satiated sooner, and so we naturally have an abundance of clean, fat-free energy to (quite literally) burn!

Eating natural fats does not spike our Insulin levels, so it cannot be converted to fatty acids and stored away in the unreachable recesses of our body.

Cold Doesn't Cause Colds

The fact that our body fat comes from ingested sugars rather than from animal fat comes as quite a shock to many people—partly because "fat" itself was also vilified by the High-Carb Pyramid, and partly because they are both inconveniently described by the same word.

By the same token, colds aren't really caused by the cold...yet this is another commonly believed myth in America.

In actual fact, cold weather *inhibits* the reproduction of germs—the colder the temperature, the fewer germs survive; that's precisely why we store our food in refrigerators and freezers. In any case, exposure to the cold stimulates and strengthens our immune system...and much more on this in an upcoming book on the benefits of cold on our bodies and waistlines.

In the end, we don't get colds in winter because it's cold outside.

We get colds in winter because we stay inside more, shake our booty less, and subsist largely on sweets and carbohydrates.

And we especially get colds when we do because up to 90% of us suffer from a Vitamin D deficiency during the winter months...which is "coincidentally" when we happen to get most of our colds!

Recall that when we cut back on excess sugars (and Mega-Sugars) we are not missing out anything useful for our beautiful bodies.

Sugars don't provide us with any value—no protein, no vitamins, no minerals, no antioxidants, no fiber. From a nutritional stand point, sugars are completely devoid of any worth.

One Step at a Time

If your goal is to weigh less, your current step is to quite deliberately begin ingesting fewer sugars.

Once more, *not* because of the calories, but because of the Insulin spike that inevitably follows.

Since this is a progression, I want you to make this lasting lifestyle change at your own pace. If your goal is to experience immediate, awe-inspiring progress in losing pounds, you may wish to cut out all excess sugars from the get-go.

That's how many of my clients do it—all at once. Or you may prefer a more gradual descent of the scale and so develop a pattern of avoiding only a single category of excess sugars at a time.

Each way is perfectly acceptable. After all, some people like to pull the Band-Aid off fast and others like to pull it off slow, and both are the right way!

If you're in the habit of eating a candy bar every afternoon, for example, the revolutionary habit-changing strategies found in Part Two will help you let go of that daily "candy bar" — or whatever other sugar-esque vice calls your name on a regular basis — and find another place to put your energies instead.

Once you become accustomed to life without the habitual afternoon candy bar, then you can take the time to examine your routine to find the *next* area where you might cut back on excess sugars.

I'm using the phrase "excess sugars" to mean stand-alone, outside sources of sugar that we eat specifically to get a sugar-rush — which we now know is actually an *Insulin-Rush.*

In other words, our goal in this progression is to cut down on sweets and donuts and ice creams, etc.

Don't yet concern yourself with ferreting out every gram of sugar from processed foods. Even if they contain sugar, go ahead and eat them...for now. (In a separate, upcoming progression, we'll target the sugars found in the manufactured foods we buy at the grocery store.)

Examples of Excess Sugars to Avoid:

Candy of all types
Sugary treats
Ice cream & gelato
Cakes & cupcakes
Pies
Donuts
Whipped cream
(Basically we're talking about candy, sweets & desserts here!)

As we've already learned, sugars aren't even the worst offenders in terms of raising our glucose levels and summoning tons of Insulin. Most of the treats made from simple sugars fall closer to the middle of the GI, while the Mega-Sugars dominate the upper reaches of the index.

But one step at a time...we'll get to the more-fattening wheat products and similar carbohydrates in due course!

Cutting Down, Cutting Back, Cutting Out

Note that Progression #2—like all the progressions—recommends that we *avoid* excess sugars, it's not insisting that we eliminate them entirely.

Let's leave the door to Christine's apartment open just a crack so our inner cat can venture out into sugar land anytime it likes. Of course, the less our inner cat goes outside, the better. Even so, do what you do without regrets.

Maintain an attitude of constant love and forgiveness for yourself—regardless of what you had for lunch or as an afternoon snack!

On the other hand, if you decide to pull the Band-Aid off quickly and let go of excess sugars entirely and permanently, then go for it.

The old adage, "Nothing tastes as good as thin feels" remains as true as ever!

But if you later decide to indulge in a piece of fudge or taffy, by all means *enjoy* it! Don't beat yourself up over anything you eat—or for any reason at all—ever again! Instead, forgive yourself and love yourself...and then get back to being Amazing!.

Even once you've discovered the secrets of how to change your habits from the inside out in Part Two, sometimes our communication channels move slowly and it can take a while for the news to travel to all the various parts of you.

In the meantime, just keep going and keep loving—

yourself, most of all!

A common argument here is, "But I have a sweet tooth"! (Which, of course, isn't an actual thing at all, but just a *habit* our body learned earlier in life.)

Nature, in her infinite wisdom, has already responded to this argument for us, since she created an entire sweet, scrumptious food category known as **fruit**.

We are allowed (encouraged, even!) to eat as much delicious fruit of any variety as we desire.

Once we cultivate the habit of enjoying fruit once again, it's often difficult to remember why we missed out on this amazing, sweet experience for so much of our lives.

So avoid excess sugars...while enjoying all the fruit you desire!

Sugar and the 'C' Word

Before we wrap up this progression, let's take our conversation about sugar one step further, because there's actually a little more to it than we've discussed so far.

Avoiding excess sugars isn't *only* about letting go of belly fat...the health implications go far beyond that.

In 2011, journalist Gary Taubes wrote an article for the New York Times Magazine with the incendiary title, *Is Sugar Toxic?*

In his oft-cited piece, Taubes says, "If sugar just makes us fatter, that's one thing. We start gaining weight, we eat less of it." But what if, Taubes asks, consuming excess sugars has a *darker* impact on our health?

How would we react if we knew that a diet heavy in sugars might also be responsible for encouraging the growth of potential cancer cells within us...or at the very least that excess sugars contribute to an environment in our bodies where cancer can grow and flourish?!

In the article, Craig B. Thompson, MD, the president of Memorial Sloan-Kettering Cancer Center explains to Taubes, "The cells of many human cancers come to depend on Insulin to provide the fuel (blood sugar) and materials they need to grow and multiply. Insulin and insulin-like growth factor also provide the signal, in effect, to do it. The more Insulin, the better the cancers do. Some cancers develop mutations that serve the purpose of increasing the influence of Insulin on the cell; others take advantage of the elevated Insulin levels that are common to metabolic syndrome, obesity and type 2 diabetes. Some do both."

In other words, Dr. Thompson believes that many pre-cancerous cells would never acquire the mutations that turn them into malignant tumors if they weren't being driven by *Insulin* to take up more and more blood sugar and metabolize it.

That's some pretty scary stuff from the highly distinguished Dr. Craig B. Thompson! So much so that the passage above probably deserves a second reading.

I'm serious, take a moment out of your life to re-read the doctor's remarks about the links between high levels of Insulin and cancer, and really take in what he's saying.

Dr. Thompson's warnings about the potential links between Insulin and cancer are worth remembering...for the rest of your life!

I should add that Craig B. Thompson, MD, isn't some "quack" from River City, Iowa with a harebrained accusation about the unproven links between refined sugars and cancer. He's the *president* of Memorial Sloan-Kettering Cancer Center in New York City — one of the most distinguished cancer research and treatment facilities in the entire world!

Dr. Thompson himself has gone even a step further than "avoiding excess sugars" that I'm recommending for you here in Progression #2.

He personally decided to *eliminate* them from his diet entirely because of the growing body of data linking sugars, excess Insulin and cancer. "I have eliminated refined sugar from my diet and eat as little as I possibly can," Dr. Thompson says, "because I believe ultimately it's something I can do to decrease my risk of cancer."

Gary Taubes concludes his brilliant write-up on the dangers of sugar in the New York Times Magazine by saying, "If it's sugar that causes insulin resistance, then the conclusion is hard to avoid that sugar causes cancer — some cancers, at least — radical as this may seem and despite the fact that this suggestion has rarely if ever been voiced before publicly."

More on the Toxicity of Sugar

You can enjoy Gary Taubes original piece, *Is Sugar Toxic?*, in its entirety by checking out this link the next time you're online.

http://www.nytimes.com/2011/04/17/magazine/mag-17Sugar-t.html?pagewanted=all

In his article, Taubes refers to another renowned medical doctor, Robert Lustig, MD — who's also something of a lone voice in the wilderness warning people about the unpublicized dangers of what he refers to as the "poison called sugar."

Dr. Lustig has become an unlikely YouTube sensation because of a talk he gave on sugar being the cause of obesity at the University of California at San Francisco a few years back because of his assertion that sugars (which necessarily include carbohydrates) cause obesity.

In an informationally dense, but always lively 90 minutes, Robert Lustig, MD, provides us with all the tested and proven science we could ever need to make a compelling case for ourselves to "avoid excess sugars" for the rest of our long and healthy lives!

Dr. Robert Lustig's presentation about the devastating effect that refined sugars have wrought upon the world in just the past 30 years is called, *Sugar: The Bitter Truth* — and has now exceeded 2 million views! You can wach the entire, life-changing lecture by going to this link on your computer:

http://www.youtube.com/watch?v=dBnniua6-oM&feature=colike

Last, and far from least, I highly recommend the book that isn't afraid to tell it like it is regarding the widespread damage that excess sugars are doing to our weight, our health and our very civilization.

SUGAR BUSTERS! by Morrison Bethea, MD, Sam Andrews, MD, Leighton Steward & Luis Balart, MD was a #1 New York Times Bestseller for good reason…it doesn't pull any punches in exposing the dangers behind the staggering 160 lbs. of refined sugar Americans consume every year.

Progression #2: Avoid Excess Sugars
YOUR NEXT STEP…

DO avoid (or eliminate, if you find the research of Dr. Thompson and Dr. Lustig sufficiently compelling!) Excess Sugars such as candy, sweets, ice cream and desserts

Do NOT worry about avoiding Excess Sugars in the processed foods you eat or the beverages you drink at this stage — we will arrive at these additional refinements in our weight-loss strategy soon enough!

*"The difference between try and
triumph is just a little umph!"*
—Marvin Phillips

PROGRESSION #3:
Avoid Wheat Products

"Don't Fill Up on Bread, Kids!"

Imagine you're a parent with the standard-issue 2.5 children (like I somehow managed to have...long story!) and you decide to take the little darlings out for dinner tonight. Doesn't matter if you're in the mood for Italian, Mexican, French, Indian, Jewish, Greek or Finnish food, chances are good the very first thing you and the kiddos will be served when you sit down at your table is *bread* in some way, shape or form.

Whether it arrives at your table in the form of rolls, pita bread, corn bread, bolillos, chips & salsa, naan bread, scones, bread sticks or any of the hundreds of white, brown or sprouted variations on that theme, bread is typically the first course at restaurants everywhere.

And not just the first course. Bread often makes up the second, fourth and even final course!

It's been estimated that wheat products, both alone in the form of bread and as part of the meal itself, account for almost *half of the entire calories consumed* during a typical restaurant visit in the United States.

After all, when we go out to a pizza place, what do we eat while waiting for the pizza (which itself is mostly bread) to finish cooking?! Many of us eat *bread sticks*, that's what!

We're basically telling the waiter, "I'll have some bread with my bread...and then gimme a side of bread

183

with that!"

Most parents have absolutely no problem whatsoever allowing their children to consume unlimited amounts of bread before, during, and after a meal.

Oh, sure, now and again one parent or another will toss out a perfunctory, "Don't fill up on bread, kids!", upon which everybody — parents included — simply nod and continue munchy-wunchying away on bread like cops at a donut-tasting convention.

After all, what's the big deal? Bread and grains are healthy for us, right?!

At the insistence of politicians who depend on Big Food's professional lobbyists to keep their re-election coffers filled, the United States Department of Carbohydrates continues to promote the heck out its new MyPlate guidelines, which *require* us maintain at least 25% of our entire food intake in the form of Insulin-producing, fat-causing breads and grains.

However, you and I finally understand the science behind how our body works — how the excess glucose from carbohydrates calls in excess Insulin to store that glucose as fat in our cells and then guard it from ever getting out again.

You and I know that breads — indeed, all products made from white flour — rank High on the Glycemic Index, in the upper 60s, while whole wheat flour scores even *higher*, in the mid 70s!

The horrific GI scores of wheat products are merely a shorthand for how much fat we store in our cells as a result of eating them. Yet eat them we do, meal after meal, because we're told to do so by career politicians — for whom old-fashioned notions like science and honesty no longer apply.

"Aside from some extra fiber, eating two slices of whole

wheat bread is really little different, and often worse, than drinking a can of sugar-sweetened soda or eating a sugary candy bar."
— Dr. William Davis

Hey Kids, Let's Fill Up on Candy!

Meanwhile, back on planet Earth, where the rest of us mere mortals are annoyingly required to obey the laws of physics and science, eating a diet high in the complex sugars known as carbohydrates causes an increase in Insulin in our bloodstream and an increase in stored fat in our cells.

At the same time, the simple sugars from the sucrose family that we are already avoiding from the previous progression actually fall closer to the middle of the Glycemic Index! Pure table sugar rates a still-high (but not carbohydrate-high!) score of 59.

The GI of a Mars bar — including nougat, chocolate, caramel and a plethora of unpronounceable chemicals — comes out at 68, basically "calling" an identical amount of fat-storing Insulin as the white bread we eat in such copious amounts. Meanwhile, the GI of a Snickers bar is only 41 — with just over *half* the Insulin-damage caused by whole wheat bread's score of 75!

Now imagine again that you've taken your little whippersnappers out to dinner. But instead of a basket of chips or bread on the table are bowls overflowing with raw sugar, each with a little spoon sticking out and a handwritten sign saying, "Eat me", in that same fancy calligraphy they always use for wedding invitations.

Also on the table are shiny platters teeming with candy bars, chocolates, truffles, fudge-cicles and pralines.

Would you encourage or even permit your children

to eat unlimited amounts of these sweets?! Of course you wouldn't. Yet we allow our children (and ourselves) to consume endless piles of wheat products at every meal—even though in terms of weight-gain, sugar damage and our overall health they are far *worse* than "merely" eating sweets!

Other than that tiny scrap of *added* Fiber (which is easily obtained from natural sources such as seeds, nuts, beans and all fruits and vegetables; in other words, *food!*) the wheat products we so promiscuously fill up on have exactly the same nutritional value as the sweets we so chastely avoid...absolutely **ZERO!**

The "Hidden Cost" of Free Bread

Have you ever wondered what's the story behind all the free bread that restaurants load us up with as soon as we walk in the door? What's in it for *them*? Why are they just giving us free stuff before we've bought anything from them yet?!

There are two reasons...

First, the Law of Reciprocity is at work here. Whenever we give somebody a present or gift of some kind, that produces in them a deep-seated desire to give something to us in return and thereby even out the balance-sheet.

One of the secrets of selling Time-Share vacation properties is the free steak dinner or even a weekend-long getaway that prospects are given.

So powerful is the prospect's desire to "return the favor" for the gift they received that they'll spend thousands of dollars or more for a vacation property they have no particular desire to ever visit.

By offering us a heaping basket of hot bread for free, restaurants are triggering the Law of Reciprocity within us and counting on us paying for all that bread and more through the increased size of our order.

Second, the heavenly *Insulin-rush* of crunchy, crunchy bread is a **powerful appetite stimulant**. Studies have shown that diners who eat bread first will order an average of 25% more food.

Earlier we learned that High-GI foods such as breads call in exceeding quantities of Insulin — which directly inhibits Leptin, the under-utilized Troubadour whose only desire is to carry a message to our body that we are full and can finally stop eating, but who gets tripped up at every turn by his arch-nemesis, Insulin.

Thanks to *receiving* the gift of bread, we feel compelled to order more food. And thanks to *eating* that free bread and spiking our Insulin levels, we feel compelled to eat all that extra food we ordered!

It's a vicious cycle that stacks the deck heavily in the favor of the restaurant, wouldn't you say?!

> *"Wheat, because of its unique blood glucose-increasing effect, makes you age faster."*
> — Dr. William Davis

Step Away From the Bread Sticks!

For most of my life, I had no idea about any of this. I mean, how would I? How would any of us?

Nobody ever sat us down in grade school — or any other school, for that matter — and explained the mechanisms of Insulin in our body and how it stored fat from excess glucose and then guarded the fat so it couldn't escape.

Heck, I always thought Insulin was just something diabetics had to take. I didn't even realize that *I* had any, much less that it was *the* critical hormone in determining how much weight I added or lost.

And nobody ever told me that the amount of excess glucose we create in our bloodstream is entirely dependent on the number of carbohydrates a food contains.

I especially never suspected that bread—whole grain, "heart healthy" bread, the food of life itself, universally endorsed by every US government "health" organization—would turn out to contain almost the highest concentration of carbohydrates that I could conceivably put in my body short of guzzling straight from a tube of High Fructose Corn Syrup!!

When I finally grasped that breads and other wheat products were among the *worst* culprits in my ongoing battle of the bulge, I was utterly floored. I didn't want to know it. I didn't want to believe it. Hey, ain't nobody what loves bread more than *this guy!*

But as I uncovered more and more truths about the severity of the damage that my ongoing consumption of breads and grains were doing to my body and belly, it finally sank in that, if anything, the increased fat buildup caused by modern wheat products is almost the *least* of it offenses.

Even so, I still kept eating bread! I still kept num-num-numming away on crackers, rolls, pasta and so on...just like all the other blissed-out-on-carbs people around me. (The main difference between us and the blissed-out Heroin addicts stumblin around downtown is they're all a lot skinnier, lulz!)

And, just like the rest of the United States, I kept getting heavier and heavier on my "healthy diet" of government-approved breads and grains.

Just Say No

For me, the straw that broke the bread stick's back came when I did my early research on the introduction of the 1992 High-Carb Pyramid and the heavy hand it seemed to play in the Obesity Nightmare that followed...a true-life horror story I shared with you above.

It was only then that I discovered there'd been many other dissenters along the way—highly respected medical doctors, nerdy scientists and too-cool-for-school journalists who for *decades* had been shouting from the mountain tops, as best they could, that the High Carb/Low Fat diet could only have one possible outcome: making us fatter than we'd ever been before. And these rabble-rousers were right.

But being *right* has no place in politics, whether you're on the Right or on the Left.

Politicians follow the money—at least the ones who intend to get re-elected do—and so these dissenting voices were studiously ignored.

In June 2011, the esteemed anti-sugar crusader, Robert Lustig, MD, gave a presentation called, "Diet, Disease and Dollars" at the MIT Club of Northern California. In his videotaped talk, Dr. Lustig—himself a distinguished MIT graduate—tells the story of meeting First Lady Michelle Obama's personal chef, Sam Kass, at a conference on obesity.

Keep in mind that Chef Sam Kass is the First Lady's point man for her Healthy Eating campaign. He sports the lofty title "Senior Policy Advisor For Healthy Food Initiatives", which Inner Beltway wags have shortened to 'Health Food Czar. '

In short, the guy's supposed to be on "our" side. In an unguarded, backstage conversation, Chef Kass told Dr. Robert Lustig that everyone on the White House staff had read Gary Taubes instant-classic New York Times Magazine piece, *Is Sugar Toxic?*, which we delved into earlier.

But Chef Kass went on to tell Dr. Lustig that *nobody* planned to do anything about the revelations in the piece.

Nobody in this—or any future—presidential

administration was going to take on Big Food directly, he said. It just wasn't gonna happen, not now, not ever.

Big Food accounts for 25% of all United States foreign exports.

Only a politician hell-bent on committing career suicide would dare call out Big Food for the hefty levels of sugars and carbohydrates they use to construct the food-shaped chemicals which line the inner aisles of grocery stores nationwide and which have plunged us into our present Obesity Nightmare. A nightmare Big Food is actively seeking to export to as many other countries as possible.

So Nero fiddled while Rome burned...and our politicians fiddle with their re-election campaigns year-round even as their constituents eat themselves quite literally to death.

The best example we could ever give to our own children is to resolve, in our own lives, never again to take dietary advice from professional lobbyists or the politicians and government organizations who answer to them. We all know that something has got to change. And it's entirely up to *us* to do the changing around here!

Listen, dude, I *know* that cutting back or cutting out the consumption of grains, pasta and other wheat products is a big, scary step to contemplate. How can we go without eating bread, for goodness sakes?!

But it's also a critical step if we truly intend to return to our natural state and our birthright of our Ideal Body.

Just hear me out on this, okay?!

Franken-Wheat

You and I already possess a hard-won understanding of the dangers from the carbohydrates in breads and grains on our waistlines.

Now let's dig deeper into some of the lesser-known health hazards of a High-Carb lifestyle and discover why wheat products in particular are something we should avoid as much as possible...even once we've returned to our Ideal Body.

It's important to understand that the wheat our great-grandparents enjoyed and the laboratory-created Franken-Wheat foisted on us today have *nothing* to do with one another. The tall, splendid amber waves of grain we still think about when we picture wheat haven't existed for some decades now. The predominant type of wheat grown in the US—indeed, the world over—is a Genetically Modified Organism (GMO) that was fabricated, quite literally, in a secret laboratory.

Called hybrid dwarf wheat, it has *less* in common genetically with the wheat our forefathers and foremothers ate than we humans do with giant sea turtles.

Like factory-produced chickens and farm-raised fish, contemporary wheat strains have been genetically modified to grow fast and furious—with two full growing cycles per annum rather than the traditional leisurely single season of the "old-fashioned" wheat. Modern wheat has become a genetic Frankenstein creation.

Oh, and think twice before you decide to enjoy one of those romantic, slow-motion runs toward your beloved through towering fields of wheat swaying in the wind that you see in all the movies!

Modern hybrid dwarf wheat barely comes up to our knees—so it's gonna look more like you're running through field of dried-up, 18" high weeds! And now for a quick reminder...

Take Advantage of the Audio Affirmations

When you're ready to implement this particular progression into your life, the Low Carb Revolution Audio Affirmations will be of enormous benefit and support to you.

The more you listen to these specially designed double-tracked affirmations, the less you'll feel cravings for bread, grains and other wheat products...so, listen to them often, my friend!

http://db.tt/69WOj7pW

Lose the Wheat, Lose the Weight

One of the world's foremost authorities on the dangers of wheat products on our collective health and waistlines is the preventative cardiologist, William Davis, MD.

His *New York Times* bestselling book, *Wheat Belly: Lose the Wheat, Lose the Wheat and Find Your Path Back to Health*, blew the lid off the poorly kept secret that wheat products cause us to gain and store more fat than even candy bars or raw sugar.

The good doctor coined the term, "Wheat Belly" to describe the dubious badge of honor that both men and women who continue to live High-Carb, bread-fueled lifestyles carry around with them on the front of their bodies 24 hours per day.

"A wheat belly represents the accumulation of fat that results from years of consuming foods that trigger Insulin, the hormone of fat storage," Dr. Davis writes.

The feisty Dr. Davis argues persuasively in *Wheat Belly* that letting go of wheat products can lead directly to improved health and the loss of the most obvious sign of our wheat addiction...our protruding wheat bellies!

The Mansierre

By any chance do you remember the classic "Seinfeld" episode where Cosmo Kramer and George Constanza's father invented the "Mansierre", a bra for guys suffering from a little too much breast development?

The episode first aired in 1994, just two years after the introduction of the High-Carb Pyramid from the USDA, and the notion of a Mansierre (or "Bro", as Kramer preferred calling it) was still side-splittingly funny back then.

Fast-forward 18 years and the punch line in a '90s sitcom has become an all-too-sad reality in America.

There are now dozens of companies actually selling "bras for men", although most of them are marketed under the less-threatening title of "compression vest" or some variation on that theme.

Now if you've ever seen seriously overweight men at the beach or pool with their protruding man-breasts you may have asked yourself why these particular men grow breasts in the first place?

Well, it's *not* because their body is selectively placing fat in such a conspicuous place on purpose to embarrass them or anything. And it's *not* that their body ran out of places to stash excess fat and their breasts were the last open frontier.

The reason for the explosion in Man Boobs in the United States has to do with...yet another hormone, what else?! (Are you beginning to see a *pattern* here? When physical changes happen to our body, a *hormone* is almost always behind that change!)

The downside of "enjoying" all-you-can-eat baskets, plates and trays of bread with every single meal is the attendant accumulation of *visceral fat*—the fat that collects around the major organs in the middle of our bodies.

Visceral fat leads to additional health complications of its own.

(NOTE: even people with moderate BMIs who appear reasonably thin and healthy on the outside can have many pounds of unseen, unhealthy *visceral fat* around the major organs of their body if they continue down the path of the High-Carb fad.)

In order to combat the inflammation of the organs caused by visceral fat, the bodies of overwheat people (ha-ha, I meant to type "overweight" people but accidentally typed "overwheat" — it made me laugh out loud when I saw it so I'm going to just leave it that way!) okay, where were we...oh yeah, visceral fat in Overwheat people (again, lulz!) leads to the production of so-called "female" hormone, Estrogen.

And it's *Estrogen* that causes increased breast growth in both obese women and men.

It's also the hormone Estrogen that causes the distinctive widening in the hips of both obese women and men...until at a certain point in time they become almost indistinguishable in appearance.

Breast-Reduction for Men

As with so many other aspects of the American Obesity Nightmare, there are plenty of opportunistic groups making quite a tidy profit from this crisis.

The fastest growing elective surgery among American men today is *Gynecosmastia* — the surgical correction of over-developed/enlarged breasts in men.

Yup, Joe Bob down the street just got his first Boob Job! (My Lord, this stuff just writes itself!)

The American Society of Plastic Surgeons are positively giddy at the unexpected profits from the influx of breast-reduction customers from the ranks of Overwheat men.

Of course, plastic surgeons don't remove the real culprit here. The visceral fat crowding out their patient's vital organs remains in place even after their reverse boob-job.

And this visceral fat just continues to accumulate as they return home from their breast-reduction surgery and resume their high-carb, high-bread lifestyle...soon producing still more Estrogen and a *return* of their dreaded man-breasts and embarrassing widened hips.

Again, visceral fat and its attendant production of the hormone Estrogen are the reason why so many overwheat—by George, I think I've coined a new word here!—men start becoming indistinguishable from women over time.

These obese men's systems are so flooded with the female-hormone Estrogen that their breasts and hips keep growing at an alarming pace...to the great confusion of the new people these men meet, who don't know whether to address them as "sir" or "madam" or something in between!

> *"For most Americans, every single meal and snack contains foods made with wheat flour. It might be the main course, it might be the side dish, it might be the dessert—and it's probably all of them."*
> —William Davis, MD

"Other Than That, Mrs. Lincoln, How Was The Play?"

And it's not just men who are suffering from the high-wheat lifestyle. The extreme, off-the-charts, Russ Meyer-esque breast sizes and double-wide hips observable in many obese women today is also caused directly by an over-production of the female hormone Estrogen in their bodies due to the accumulation of visceral fat around their vital organs.

If the *only* benefit from avoiding wheat products was to help us slow the growth of misshapen bodies from Estrogen overload and to help us lose the accumulations of visceral fat around our major organs, that alone would make it a completely worthwhile endeavor.

But we're still just at the tip of the iceberg of the harm that ubiquitous wheat products are doing to our collective health.

William Davis, MD, has done us the good service of writing an entire, highly readable book called *Wheat Belly* on the health consequences of over-consuming breads and grains.

Rather than spend page after page summarizing Dr. Davis' well-documented research and compelling case histories, I'm going to strongly recommend you seek out and read his book yourself.

Here are just a couple of highlights — or lowlights, depending on your perspective! — that you can expect to learn from reading *Wheat Belly*:

The effect of wheat products on the precipitous rise and dramatic fall in blood sugar levels creates an almost morphine-like addiction to it

Wheat products are appetite stimulants — the more you eat, the more you want

Celiac Disease: the only known cure for this health-threatening illness is to eliminate gluten (a key component of wheat products and the stuff that makes dough all stretchy and knead-y) from your diet entirely.

Studies show that elimination of wheat products alone leads to a *natural* reduction in total daily caloric intake by 350-400 calories...and having a lower caloric intake is a universal predictor of longevity.

Cholesterol levels improve markedly with the elimination of wheat products from the diet

Wheat products cause high amounts of what are known as Advanced Glycation End-Products (AGE) — which promote aging in our bodies, form wrinkles, lead to loss of skin elasticity, the growth of cataracts and even contribute to dementia. (In short, consumption of wheat products makes us look and feel old!)

Wheat Belly

Back when I still weighed close to 270 pounds, not only did I consume bread with virtually every meal like the rest of the inmates, I also learned how to bake bread and took no small pride in hand-crafting one or several ginormous loafs of bread each week. So, again, I'm definitely a man what loves himself some bread!

Hell, I even kept the classic bread-making cookbook by Edward Espe Brown, *The Tassajara Bread Book* (known popularly as "The bible for bread baking"!) on my nightstand so I could page through it at night and fantasize about the exotic loaves of bread I would one day bake.

Therefore it was with a very heavy heart indeed when I finally realized that bread and I were always going to have an utterly dysfunctional relationship — and that I was never going to regain my health and lose my wheat belly until I lost the wheat itself.

And that's when I ultimately made the tough decision that bread and I were just gonna have to break up and go our separate ways.

When you get to that point in your relationship with wheat products, Dr. William Davis' gripping tome about the litany of health and weight dangers caused by wheat products can help make your own decision to break up with bread a whole lot easier, lemme tell ya!

I highly recommend you pick up a copy of *Wheat Belly*. Read it and then decide for yourself if you want to take this important plunge in your life to avoid wheat products in order to improve your health and reduce your waistline.

As Dr. Davis eloquently puts it, "What have you got

to lose except your wheat belly, your man breasts, or your bagel butt?"

Or as I put it—"Every Overwheat person in America should read *Wheat Belly*!"

The Matrix is All Around Us

Let's remind ourselves why we are here. Ostensibly it's to lose weight. And, yes, for sure, we're making great progress in that direction both in our understanding of how our bodies gain and store fat and in what we can specifically do to turn that around.

But there's *another* reason we're on this journey, if you recall.

You and I have been brought together ultimately to help wake up your *Inner Self*—that highest, most powerful part of you that's been slumbering deep inside you for years and years now.

It is my considered belief that it was the effect on our blood glucose from all the sugars and Mega-Sugars we consumed when we were younger that caused this highest part of us to "go to sleep" in the first place.

And it is my even stronger belief that a critical step in the process of *waking up to our true Potential* is to let go of the carbohydrates and the pastas and the breads that have been keeping us asleep.

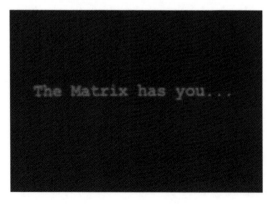

One of the reasons why the sci-fi movie *The Matrix* became such a worldwide success was that audiences everywhere recognized that they, too, were *asleep* on some level, and they would never be free until they figured out how to wake up and join the world of the living.

What if I'm right?! What if wheat products and other high-carbohydrate "foods" are keeping us asleep?

If we had to pick between waking up and continuing to sleep our life away, which would we choose? Would we choose to eat scrumptious, mouth-watering, munchy-crunchy bread with each meal and sleep through life, as so many of us do...or would we choose to finally *live* our dreams?

Would we decide to have another poppy seed bagel...or write the Great American Novel? Should we scarf down that extra-large bag of sea-salt-encrusted, butterfly-shaped pretzels...or go have the most conscious, transformative sex of our entire lives? Do we order the Bottomless Bowl of Pasta...or enjoy the feeling of a beautiful body teeming with awareness, energy and life?

Only *you* have the answers to these questions.

Recall that a superior strategy for making decisions is to spend time in front of the Altar of You that you created earlier...and ask, "If I truly loved myself, what would I choose here?"

And then go in the direction that your beautiful body, your loving heart and your awakening Inner Self point you!

Progression #3: Avoid Wheat Products
YOUR NEXT STEP...

DO avoid wheat products as much as possible

Do NOT replace wheat products with traditional "Gluten-Free" products, which often contain the only known foodstuffs that score *higher* on the Glycemic Index than breads and grains: starches. (NB: Gluten-Free foods created from tapioca starch, rice starch, corn starch and the like are even worse for our health and weight than wheat products!)

> *"People who eliminate wheat from their diet typically report improved mood, fewer mood swings, improved ability to concentrate, and deeper sleep within just days to weeks of their last bite of bagel or baked lasagna."*
> — William Davis, MD

PROGRESSION #4:
Drink Alcohol in Moderation

The Proverbial Last 10 Pounds

You can totally skip this progression if you want. Seriously, I have no intentions of standing directly in the path between you and your alcoholic beverage(s) of choice.

All I ask is that you read this chapter first and then decide for yourself how much or how little you want to continue drinking in the future.

That's a reasonable enough request, no?! And by way of incentive to get you to actually *consider* these ideas, I want you to know that this progression is where the proverbial Last 10 Pounds are to be found...or *lost*, as the case may be!

When you get to the juncture where you have a decision to make about whether or not you want to do whatever it takes to lose those Last 10 Pounds, at that point reducing the amount of alcohol you drink will become more important.

Believe me, at first I didn't want to know the truth about how alcohol directly impacted my weight, just as once upon a time I didn't want to know that the cause of my former wheat belly was largely bread itself!

But it's called the *truth* for a reason, so let's cozy up to the bar, order a stiff one and examine the role of alcohol in our bodies!

A Calorie By Any Other Name...

Calories are units of potential energy that our bodies can convert into glucose and then burn off as needed. As a general rule, calories are not our enemy. The fat stored in our bodies does not come from ingesting more calories, it comes entirely from eating foods rich in sugars and carbohydrates which score high on the Glycemic Index.

Even so, the calories we take in *do* need to be burned up first before we can begin using the reserves of energy stored in our liver and other parts of our bodies as glycogen (immediately usable energy) and fat (stored energy).

The good news about alcohol — and by "alcohol" I mean distilled spirits such as Scotch, whiskey, vodka, gin, tequila, mescal and the like — is that because of the distillation process it is both carbohydrate-free and gluten-free.

Meanwhile, wine and beer are *fermented* rather than distilled, so wine contains carbohydrates, while wheat-based beers contain both carbohydrates and gluten. We'll come back to wine and beer in a bit, but for now when I refer to "alcohol" I'm speaking of distilled spirits.

Again, the good news: no carbs and no gluten in any alcohol.

The bad news: calories...and lots of them! Alcohol contains 7 calories per gram — nearly twice as much as the 4 calories in carbohydrates or protein, and not too far below fat, with 9 calories per gram.

There are close to 100 calories in a single, one-ounce shot of liquor. The large 1.75 liter bottle of booze that's so popular today contains approximately 64 ounces...or the equivalent of 64 shots.

Let's do the math together: 64 ounces x 100 calories

= 6400 calories in a standard large bottle sold at liquor stores.

Any way you slice it that's a fair number of calories for our body to process and which we will need to burn off as energy before we can get back to using the energy reserves we already have stored in our bodies.

Burn, Baby, Burn!

For most of my adult life I drank almost every evening. Not enough to get falling down drunk, but I enjoyed a good buzz as much as anybody.

Because of my size—6'3", 189 lbs.—it took more than a couple of drinks to get that buzz on, and I eventually developed the habit of drinking about two bottles of liquor (Scotch primarily, in case you wondered!) each week. Let's get some more math out of the way…

64 ounces per bottle x 100 calories per ounce = 6400 calories per bottle of alcohol

2 bottles x 6400 calories = 12,800 extra calories per week in liquidious form that I was taking in

According to the Caloric Weight Gain Myth you have to either eat or burn approximately 3500 calories in order to gain or lose a pound, respectively.

If that Myth were true, I would have necessarily gained over 3.5 lbs per week from my alcohol consumption alone!

And with 52 weeks in a year, the Caloric Weight Gain Myth would require me to have gained 190 lbs. in a single year, which is equivalent to a whole other me— and that's supposing that all of the rest of my food intake resulted in an exact energy balance!

Although the Calories In, Calories Out dogma pounded into us since our youth has proved to be not just wrong, but laughably so, our bodies still *do* need to burn off any excess energy sources before it can return to using up our stored fat.

In other words, I wasn't any storing much if any fat because of the alcohol calories I was taking in. Those calories were being burned off as fast as my body could reasonably do so.

Yet, at the same time, I went through an endless period of what's referred to colloquially as a "weight loss stall", during which time I lost no additional weight despite running an otherwise pretty tight ship in terms of good eating habits.

No wonder I couldn't ever quite lose those Last 10 Pounds despite already following every other progression of the *Low Carb Revolution* — almost 13,000 additional calories per week to burn off is no trivial number!

Even though calories most definitely do not count on a pound-to-pound ratio — everybody other than Big Diet knows that 3500 calories do NOT actually cause us to gain or lose exactly one pound! — calories do count a little bitty bit, and we can't be completely unmindful of them. We'll talk more about calories in just a few moments..

Only when I cut back from drinking every single night did I finally lose the Last 10 Pounds — which I've easily kept off ever since through my ongoing healthy lifestyle.

"A Little Extra"

That said, not everybody necessarily wants to lose those Last 10 Pounds.

I personally take no small pride in having the lean body of a triathlete without the any of the inconvenience and hard work of actually training for and competing in triathlons!

For me losing the Last 10 Pounds was just a fun game I wanted to play with my body in order to discover how it looked and felt to return to the exact same weight I enjoyed as a teenager in high school.

Although it would certainly be possible for me to drop even lower, I have no desire to do so, since there are no health advantages in being excessively thin. Quite the opposite, in fact! Being too skinny creates health drawbacks of its own accord.

For the purposes of longevity—in other words, living a long-ass time—the ideal body type to aspire towards involves a return to a boring, "normal" weight for our height and age...and then what's referred to as "a little extra."

Statistically, people with just a little cushion on top of a normal body weight live longer, healthier lives than people who weigh substantially less or more.

That's why, unlike any of the other progressions, there's more inherent flexibility in this particular strategy.

And even then, remember I'm not insisting that you "avoid" alcohol entirely, but rather drink in perhaps more moderation than you've been accustomed to doing previously.

You *can* decide to avoid alcohol completely...or very nearly so. Or you can simply cut back on your alcohol consumption...yet still enjoy a moderate level of drinking if you choose.

How The Body Burns Alcohol

The problem with alcohol isn't limited to its astronomical calorie count, but also with the way our bodies *process* those calories.

Unlike the calories from the other three substances our bodies recognize as sources of energy (protein, fats and carbohydrate), the calories from alcohol are treated in a completely different fashion, which creates tribulations of its own.

205

When alcohol enters our body, it is given a red-carpet, First-Class treatment. It goes straight to the head of the line of *any other* foods or drinks we were already processing.

Now this isn't because our bodies consider alcohol to be the Coolest Kid on the Block, worthy of VIP treatment.

Quite the contrary — alcohol is considered to be a *poison* by our bodies, and that's why it makes every effort to process it and get it the hell out of us as soon as possible!

Our liver is the only organ in our body that can process alcohol — and it does so at the relatively modest rate of 1 oz. (the equivalent of that 100-calorie single shot) per hour. Our liver converts the alcohol into a substance called acetate, which brings us to another good news/bad news fork in the road.

The Good News: acetate itself is not readily stored as fat in our cells.

The Bad News: the acetate still has to be burned off before our body turns to other energy sources to power us through our activities.

When we're drinking, our body relies entirely and exclusively on the energy from the calories in the alcohol before it gives our heroic hormone Glucagon the okay to start liberating our stored fats and burn them off.

The Munchies

Alcohol produces another undesirable side-effect in our systems. You may recall how restaurant owners absolutely love it when their patrons start right in eating bread when they sit down at the table because the bloodsugar/Insulin-rush from the carbohydrates stimulates their appetite and leads to greater quantities of food being ordered and consumed.

Restaurant owners' *second*-favoritist thing in the

world is when customers also order an alcoholic beverage before deciding on their entree—because drinking alcohol leads to larger orders still.

Research has shown there's a *20% increase in caloric intake* in the form of food when alcohol is consumed during a meal…and a *total caloric boost of 33%* when the calories from alcohol are added into the mix!

That's a pretty staggering amount of additional of calories to load up on at a single meal, wouldn't you say?!

This is the reason why restaurants usually do their utmost to get an alcoholic beverage in you at the earliest possible moment, sometimes even hiring a dedicated cocktail server whose sole job is to expedite the process and get a little buzz going on in your system before you ever place your order.

And it's de rigeur at those fancy restaurants where the shiny people dine that the waiter won't even come around to take your order until you're starting in on your second round of drinks.

Now the reason why we devour fully one-third more calories while drinking liquor during a meal is because of alcohol's direct influence on two very important hormones we've already been introduced to…

Ghrelin—our Inner Troubadour who bears the urgent message that we're hungry and it's high time for us to eat something.

&

Leptin—the Troubadour who is supposed to let us know we are full and can now stop eating, but whose job is all too often derailed by the actions of thuggish hormones like Insulin and Ghrelin, both of which are fond of kidnapping Leptin and tying it to a chair in the sub-basement of our bodies and playing the soundtrack of *Reservoir Dog*s while preventing it from delivering its

"I'm full now stop eating" message.

Because it *stimulates* the hormone Ghrelin and *inhibits* the hormone Leptin, alcohol creates a negative double-whammy within us that makes it nearly physiologically impossible to resist consuming any available food sources once we begin drinking.

Hungry Like A Wolf

We previously learned that Ghrelin is the nagging hormone that drives us to eat by making us all grumpy and cranky and shiz until we put something (anything!) in our stomachs.

Drinking alcohol causes a surge of Ghrelin in our system, which produces an overwhelming biological drive to seek out food in some form or another.

As if alcohol's soaring count of 7 calories per gram wasn't enough, alcohol also drives us to consume even more calories under its influence.

This is the reason why drinking gives us the "munchies" — that almost irresistible compulsion to put additional food in our system regardless of its nutritional value or lack thereof.

Alcohol makes us hungry by motivating the secretion of Ghrelin. Yet our "hunger hormone" also has a couple of additional messages it likes to deliver on the side...neither of which are messages we particularly want our body to hear.

Bonus Communication #1 from Ghrelin concerns what we should *do* with any food we eat under its influence — and the gist of the message is that we should store that food as fatty acids in our gut.

Dr. Amaia Rodriguez Murueta-Goyena (now that's a mouthful!) describes the process, "The Ghrelin hormone not only stimulates the brain, giving rise to an increase in appetite, but also favors the accumulation of lipids in visceral fatty tissue, located in the abdominal zone and considered to be most harmful."

In other words, Ghrelin makes us hungry *and* causes us to store whatever food we eat directly as visceral fat in our bellies.(Which, again, is the worst place for it...since visceral fat causes *inflammation* in our organs and also leads to the excess Estrogen production that's making everybody's boobs and hips expand like a blow-up doll from a novelty store.)

Just as with Insulin, we generally want to avoid "calling" Ghrelin as much as possible...because, frankly, no good can from it under normal circumstances.

As we progress further along the *Low Carb Revolution* lifestyle and take in a greater percentage of energy-dense proteins and fats from both plants and animals, we will feel more satiated from morning til night and Ghrelin will rarely need to rouse itself from its heavy slumbers to make the rounds in our system.

And that's just the way we want it! Because *Ghrelin is not our friend!* It has nothing of value to offer our bodies and the less it hangs around, the better!

This is why we don't want to allow ourselves to become overly hungry, even when we're not drinking, because the natural result of severe hunger is to call in Ghrelin to induce us to eat.

People who still follow the calorie-counting fad often report feeling hungry "almost all the time". As a result, their system is constantly awash in Ghrelin, which is trying to compel them to eat some damn food for a change!

Because of the continuous presence of Ghrelin in their bloodstream, the meager amount of food these famished, calorie-counting dieters *do* allow to pass their impoverished lips is stored preferentially as visceral fat in their bellies.

Maybe you've known people like this—who

consume an insanely low number of calories each day on one of those horried calorie-counting diets, and yet still continue to add fat and weight despite their meager eating habits.

Well, it was Ghrelin, the hunger-hormone activated by their reduced-calorie diet, that caused this perfect storm of fat build-up in their bodies.

Even among people who eat healthy amounts of actual food, alcohol can still trigger the Ghrelin response—leading to hunger and the build-up of unwanted visceral fat.

As if increasing our appetite and building abdominal fat wasn't enough, researchers have recently discovered that Ghrelin has yet *another* message that contributes to the alcohol-hunger-alcohol feedback loop.

Bonus Communication #2 from Ghrelin involves stimulating the structures in our brain associated with pleasure-seeking and reward.

Here's how it works...Ghrelin targets the "reward centers" of our brain, which in turn stimulates us to drink more alcohol so that more Ghrelin will be called and we'll feel even better, which calls still more Ghrelin!

So the feedback loop now looks like this...

Alcohol -> Ghrelin -> Pleasure ->
More Alcohol -> More Ghrelin -> More Pleasure ->
Hunger -> Eat Krap -> Gain Visceral Fat
(REPEAT CYCLE ad infinitum)

One of the reasons why it's often so difficult for heavy drinkers to give up the booze is because the Ghrelin called in by their drinking activates the structures of their brains associated with *reward*.

In turn this spurs an almost overpowering desire for future alcohol consumption...not just at a single-sitting, but over the long-haul.

In other words, the brains of heavy drinkers "remember" how good it felt the last time they drank and it actively encourages them to drink yet more of alcohol so the brain can enjoy that pleasurable reward response once again.

Renowned researcher into the links between Ghrelin and obesity, Dr. Suzanne Dickson notes: "Ghrelin's actions in the brain may be of importance for all kinds of addictions, including chemical drugs such as alcohol and even food."

But stimulating Ghrelin is just the first half of the one-two punch that alcohol delivers to our hormones.

Get Thee Behind Me, Leptin!

We're already well-acquainted with our under-utilized Inner Troubadour known as Leptin. Straight up: alcohol consumption also inhibits our appetite-suppressing hormone Leptin.

According to Dr. Jan Calissendorff, "A moderate amount of alcohol induces a significant inhibition of both diurnal and nocturnal secretion of Leptin."

Even after giving in to our biological hunger cravings and scarfing down a huge, carb-heavy midnight snack after an evening of drinking, when we wake up the next morning we still feel hungrier than usual and are driven to eat yet more food on top of our usual morning fare.

To recap: drinking alcohol calls Ghrelin, which makes us hungry and also stimulates the *reward-response* centers of our brain, which strongly prefers that we satisfy that hunger with sugary carbohydrates that will give us a blissful Insulin-rush.

Then because of the absence of Leptin, once we do start eating under the influence of alcohol, we just keep on eating and keep on eating, far past the point of our immediate energy needs.

And recall that because our system usually doesn't store the calories from alcohol but instead burns them as energy as quickly as possible, in truth we have no immediate energy needs while we are drinking!

You could almost say it's a malfunction of our system that causes us to become physically hungry and consume even more food while drinking alcohol, except for the rather significant fact that drinking alcohol is not a normal or natural thing for the human body to do in the first place.

There's nothing wrong with our internal systems—they work just fine! However, our body did not evolve to process alcohol, and considers it a toxin to get rid as hurriedly as possible.

A toxin that, alas, has some undesirable and yet unavoidable side effects, as we've just learned.

Beer and Wine

The conversation has centered entirely on liquor up until now, so let's briefly touch on two other categories of alcoholic beverages: Beer and Wine.

Both possess the same negative side-effects...calling in the hunger-causing, abdominal-fat-creating hormone Ghrelin and suppressing the I'm-Full-You-Can-Stop-Eating-Now hormone Leptin.

BEER:

As you surely already know or at least strongly suspect, beer is a double-whammy of non-goodness. Beer contains carbohydrates, or Mega-Sugars in abundance—leading to the highly sexy (in Pretend World!) *beer belly*.

Additionally, most popular beers also contain gluten from the wheat it was brewed from, which has its own negative impacts on our health.

(If you still haven't checked out Dr. William Davis' excellent volume on how modern-day Franken-wheat became a significant contributor to our collective Obesity Nightmare, you owe it your waistline and your health to look into *Wheat Belly*.)

Beer not only has the expected 100 calories per ounce of alcohol, it also has moderate to high levels of carbohydrates—which instantly spike our blood sugar and cause that old, familiar, blissful Insulin-rush which causes fat storage in our cells.

I'm a native Texan and beer is what we drink in the great state of Texas. Beer is what I drank for many, many years.

But long before I generally weaned myself off alcoholic beverages, I specifically switched over from consuming beer to distilled spirits in order to cut down on all the sugary carbohydrates.

If your ultimate goal is to return to your Ideal Weight, I would strongly recommend you consider doing the same. All you need to remember is that *beer is nothing more than Liquid Bread!*

WINE:

If you enjoy drinking, most researchers suggest that wine remains the most healthiest choice. Although wine does contain carbohydrates, they're low in number compared to beer. And there are numerous studies showing that drinking moderate amounts of wine can have a positive impact on our health, especially when it comes to anti-oxidants.

Writers like Timothy Ferriss (who brought us such gems as the *Four-Hour Work Week* and the *Four-Hour Body*) have shown that it's possible to maintain a super low body fat percentage and a sick set of six-pack abs while still consuming a couple of glasses of red wine on a nightly basis!

So, drink beer as little as possible, and wine in moderation.

Oh, and don't just drink wine in moderation, drink any and all alcoholic beverages in moderation.

Now the calories and such we've been discussing so far in distilled spirits hasn't even been taking into consideration all the sugary juices, mixers and tonics that tend to accompany modern mixed drinks. And it's *these* liquid sugars and Mega-Sugars that can quickly take our glucose levels through the roof and summon our old bugaboo, Insulin.

Blame It On the Mi-Mi-Mi-Mixers!

When it comes to alcoholic drinks and our worn down, overworked, under-appreciated inner Troubadour known as Insulin, the real culprit comes in the form of Mixers.

Other than straight soda water—which is fairly harmless and sugar-free—virtually every other mixer we add to our alcoholic beverages contains heaps of sugars and Mega-Sugars, and therefore should only be used in considered moderation.

Mixers can include the sugary, off-the-shelf stuff found at liquor stores…or simply tippling a splash of artificial fruit juice into our drinks. All too often these additional sugars are hiding in plain sight and we don't even consider them when making or ordering a drink.

Fancy and exotic drinks almost always contain high levels of added sugars and Mega-Sugars from their mixers.

As a general rule, if it's served in a coconut or has a colorful paper umbrella sticking out of it, you can guarantee your Insulin is in for a bumpy night!

If we can find ways to cut back or cut down on the sweetened Mixers we put into our drinks, then losing excess weight can increasingly become a reality for us.

Even if we implement every other suggested progression in the Low Carb Revolution lifestyle but still continue to drink sugary, sweetened alcoholic beverages on a regular basis, our progress will be slow and our weight loss can become stalled.

Liquor versus Liqueur

Liquor is just another name for distilled beverages — all of which have 0 carbohydrates and are gluten-free regardless of the grain they were distilled from.

Liqueur, on the other hand, refers to alcoholic beverages to which sugar and other sweet flavorings have been added. Liqueurs include sweet drinks such as Grand Marnier, Schnapps, Kahlua, Amaretto, Triple Sec and so on. Liqueurs do contain carbohydrates — and lots of them — and therefore should be avoided or consumed very sparingly.

Wait, I Thought Calories Didn't Matter?!

In the second half of the *Low Carb Revolution* I'm going to make a strong case that our "problems" cannot be solved by *thinking* about them...that the usefulness of our brains in overcoming our internal obstacles, fears and wounds has been ridiculously over-stated.

Even though I deliberately under-exaggerate the brain's potential ability to help improve our lives, I'm not saying that our Mind has ZERO impact on improving our lives. Our mind just has far less impact on our decisions and habits than we've been led to believe.

Bottom line: the sooner we get out of our Head and into our Body, the sooner real change and transformation can take place.

Similarly, throughout the book so far I've been making poopy all over the Caloric Myth of Weight

Loss, in no small part because it is demonstrably false in my life, your life, and the lives of everyone who ever subjected themselves to a reduced-calorie diet.

Not eating 3500 calories over the course of one or more days does not directly result in losing a pound of weight...nor does eating 3500 calories over any particular period of time lead inescapably to our gaining a pound of weight.

Yet, at some considerably, smaller, lower, less-than-we've-been-told level calories *do* factor into the equation. A little.

Even though I did not gain 3.5 pounds per week (or a total of 190 pounds per year) by drinking upwards of 12,800 calories in alcohol alone each week, I still never lost the legendary Last 10 Pounds until I stopped loading up my body with all those unnecessary calories.

As soon as I cut well back on my drinking, the Last 10 Pounds vanished like dropping a chocolate eclair on an ant hill!

The hapless few people who actually manage to suffer through an entire year of restricting themselves by the appointed 1000 calories per day below their normal energy needs do not, of course, ever lose the combined 365,000 calories (1000 calories x 365 days) worth of weight that the Caloric Weight Loss Myth hypothesizes.

This would amount to a staggering total weight loss of **104 pounds** in a single year and every obese human alive would therefore already be on a restricted calorie diet and we wouldn't need this book or any other to tell us how to eat, right?!

Nobody in the history of calorie counting ever lost the 104 pounds that creating a daily, thousand-calorie deficit should inescapably lead to...or anything close to that number.

Numerous studies at the 12-month mark show the average weight loss for the most popular restricted-calorie diet on the market today is in the range of 6-8 pounds.

By withholding *365,000 total calories* from their food consumption over a year, their paltry net loss of calories stored as fat in their body ranges from 21,000 (6 lbs.) to 31,500 (9 lbs.)

On the one hand, we might ask, "Where did the other 333,000+ calories that they *didn't lose* go?! What happened to that 1/3 of a million calories that *they didn't eat and yet didn't lose*...and why are they still hanging around on their waistline?!"

But on the other hand, we might ask a more pointed question: "How did they manage to lose *any* weight on a calorie-counting regime?!"

Losing 6-8 pounds instead of shedding the predicted *104 pounds* of this restricted calorie diet is hardly an impressive tipping of the scales by any measure, but that's not the point here.

Our takeaway is that these poor restricted-calorie victims did not lose ZERO weight!

In other words, while their draconian restriction of calories did not result in an equally memorable loss of weight, it did lead to *some* small weight loss, which means that we should at least pay some small—*very small*—attention to the overall calories we consume.

It's not surprising that a massive campaign of calorie-counting doesn't lead to spectacular weight loss, what *is* surprising is that it leads to *any* weight loss whatsoever! (Of course, it's also quite possible—and even likely—that even the 6-8 pounds that hardcore calorie counters are able to shed over the year can be explained entirely by **the Hawthorne Effect**, which we'll discover later.)

In any case, the high calorie count of 7 calories per

gram in alcohol, as well as its debilitating impact on our Master Hormone Leptin—which pioneers such as Dr. Jack Kruse argue is the key hormone in our entire energy system—was the primary reason why I decided to limit my alcohol intake somewhat...and it's the reason I'm encouraging you to consider doing the same!

Progression #4: Drink Alcohol in Moderation
YOUR NEXT STEP...

DO avoid beer because of its carbohydrate and gluten content

DO drink wine in moderation

DO drink distilled spirits in moderation

DO avoid drinking alcohol *during a meal* unless your specific goal is to order and consume greater quantities of food...like if you're trying to eat one of those whole 72-ounce steaks so you can get it for free and get your picture on the wall!

DO be aware that the more we drink, the more of the appetite-stimulating hormone Ghrelin will be called in, which causes us to become increasingly hungry and also stores the ingested calories directly as belly fat

DO avoid Mixers—which are largely sugars and carbs in liquid form

DO avoid sweetened Liqueurs

DO add a twist of lemon or lime to "de-acidify" your drinks (see the Progression on pH below)

"The body generally utilizes alcohol as an immediate source of energy. While doing this, the body will not burn any energy from body reserves (fat!)."
—Morrison Bethea, MD, Sam Andrews, MD, Leighton Steward & Luis Balart, MD in *SUGAR BUSTERS!*

PROGRESSION #5:
Avoid Processed Carbs

The 80/20 Rule

According to the 80/20 Rule (referred to by know-it-all economists as the "Pareto principle"), for a great many events approximately 80% of our results will come from only 20% of our actions.

We're going to continue to add a few more distinctions that will take us further down the road towards our goal of returning to our birthright and natural state of our Ideal Body. Yet in terms of actual dietary changes we're going to make together, the progressions we've already covered easily account for 80% of all the "work" in store for us.

If we can successfully create new habits in our lives where we simply avoid excess sugars, avoid wheat products and drink alcohol in moderation, then we'll already have done most of the heavy lifting.

Each of the remaining progressions offers smaller, more discrete steps on our journey of transforming ourselves from the inside out.

Continue to go at your own pace here. If you're more comfortable spending weeks or longer adjusting your body to lower amounts of excess sugars or wheat products before moving on to the next progression, that is exactly what you should do. Our goal at all times is to recreate ourselves and *wake up* at a pace where we always feel safe, protected and loved.

And recall that I've given you an additional, free tool to assist you in exactly those areas. The *Low Carb Revolution* audio affirmations were carefully designed to create powerful, positive messages for your Mind and Body that will help you rewrite an entirely new story in you life...and do so in an environment where you can feel completely *supported*.

Play these audio affirmations in the background as often as possible to keep delivering these important message to yourself. *They really will help you make this new lifestyle easier and more sustainable!*

http://db.tt/69WOj7pW

Also, if you have any questions, feedback, or success stories, please feel free to contact me any time at my personal email address: **zombiejohn@gmail.com**.

Put "Low Carb Revolution" somewhere in the message header to make sure your note doesn't languish as possible spam in my inbox.

Carbs Are Not Our Friend

Let's get right to the point of this Progression. In a nutshell...

Avoid processed Mega-Sugars.

Recall that Mega-Sugars is my cheeky name for the sachharides that Big Food/Big Diet reverently refers to carbohydrates.

Glossy magazines promoting "athletic lifestyles", as well as makers of sugary "sports" drinks and career politicians who depend on lobbyist $$$ for re-election have hijacked the term "carbohydrates" and put it on an altar. And we are commanded to worship their Carbohydrate God on a daily basis.

But I've come along—as others before me have come along—to remind good people such as yourself that the Carbohydrate God is a false god and should not be worshipped.

Quite the opposite. Carbohydrates are not our friend.

Carbohydrates score near the top of the Glycemic Index, an indication of how much glucose any particular food will introduce into our bloodstream.

Carbohydrates spike our blood sugar off the chart, which then calls in a flood of Insulin to store all that excess glucose as fat and guard it from escaping. Carbohydrates cause us to gain weight and maintain that weight. Carbohydrates are not food. They are not required to sustain human life—only Protein, Fat and Fiber are.

"Carbohydrates" is the popular, advertiser-friendly name for the family of complex sugars better known to scientists as saccharides, or Mega-Sugars, as I refer to them. *Carbohydrates do one thing and one thing only for us: they make us fat.*

To sum up my mini-rant, the state-mandated worship of the Carbohydrate God has, in a mere twenty years, turned the United States of America into the most obese nation in the history of the world…and it's just getting worse.

Time to *Defriend* Carbs

If you're a member of Facebook, you've probably had more than one occasion to Defriend a particular obnoxious or boorish person on your Friend list. I think it's high time we Defriend carbohydrates. More specifically, for this particular progression, we're going to Defriend *processed* carbs.

There are certain natural foods—a very few fruits and a very few vegetables—that are also high in carbohydrates and therefore cause us to call excess Insulin that will create and store excess fat. But that's the subject of a future progression. We're not gonna worry our pretty little heads about any *naturally* occurring carbs for now!

Instead, our focus is on avoiding *processed* Mega-Sugars. How do we know where these carbs are? Well, they generally hide out in a particularly insidious substance that humans consume on all-too-regular basis. A substance I have termed...

Food-Shaped Chemicals

All the real food in a typical American grocery store can be found along the outer ring: fruits, vegetables, meats, fish, poultry and dairy.

The interior aisles of grocery stores consist largely of what I refer to as **food-shaped chemicals** — processed concoctions of artificial ingredients which are always high in carbohydrates, the very things we want to avoid if our goal is to let go of the fat stored in our bodies.

These products are created (quite literally) in laboratories from a Frankenstein-ish combination of wheat, corn, soy, and real or artificial sweeteners...and then sprinkled liberally with unpronounceable chemicals designed to make them more palatable and/or to give them a shelf-life that will far outlast the hapless consumers they were designed for.

Food-shaped chemicals can also be found at your local McTacoHut — where the "meat" in your burger or taco regularly contains less than 33% of anything actually resembling meat. (Most Fat Food products are made up mostly of corn, wheat and soy fillers, with just enough "meat" or "chicken" thrown in to avoid prosecution under the letter of the law...all of which is held together by a particularly unctuous substance known within the industry as "Meat Glue"!)

Pop quiz: What percentage of Chicken McNugget is actually chicken?

Not only are these food-shaped chemicals not food, they are exceedingly high in carbohydrates and thus contribute directly to our ongoing Obesity Nightmare.

Answer to Pop Quiz: According to Michael Pollan's book, *The Omnivore's Dilemma*, a mere **18%** of the McNugget is truly chicken. The rest is a slurry of cheap, fattening carbohydrates held together with the ubiquitous you-REALLY-don't-wanna-know-what's-in-it Meat Glue!

Now I'm not going to present you with a laundry list of foods high in processed carbohydrates for you to avoid, not least since that list would contain many thousands of items that in the past we mistook for food.

And even then, would you really carry that list around and consult it every time you made a food purchase? Instead I want to help you become a more informed and aware food consumer.

Here are some general guidelines to get you started. I invite you to start asking a few questions whenever you're in the grocery store selecting an item.

Does the product you are considering purchasing contain sugars or wheat flour?

Is the product high in carbohydrates?

Does the product contain 5 or more ingredients?

Does the product contain nutritional information based on an unrealistic number of servings per package (such as for .65 piece of a candy bar package that contains two pieces of candy!)

Does it come in packaging that looks like it was designed for Soviet astronauts to squeeze out in a zero-gravity environment?

But most of all...does the product have lots of carbohydrates?

If you answered "yes" to any of these questions, then the item you are holding in your hand is most likely a product to be *avoided* rather than actual food to be enjoyed!

Do The Math!

Another ruse to watch out for is Big Food trying to trick you with unrealistic serving sizes. Manufacturers are required by law to list ingredients, nutrition data and carbohydrates on their packaging...but there's a lot of "play" in these requirements.

For example, the required information can be listed according to each *serving* of the item in question. Commonly these servings are in no way representative of what a real human being would actually eat...such as when a tiny cardboard container with 6 ounces of juice claims to contain, "2.5 servings."

Big Food and its wholly owned subsidiary, Big Diet, are *counting* on the fact that we're not gonna do the math ourselves.

Recently I stumbled upon an online site selling Atkins candy. (Why in the world a company that supposedly promotes weight loss actively manufactures and sells sweets is another conversation entirely.) This particular candy was basically Atkins' version of the popular Reese's Peanut Butter Cup.

When I checked the number of Mega-Sugars in the candy, they seemed rather high to me at 18 carbohydrates.

But then something caught my eye: the amount of servings. This one little package of just two chocolatey peanut butter cups was listed as **5 servings!**

Seriously, is there any human alive, overweight or not, on planet Earth who would take *5 separate sittings to consume two tiny peanut butter cups?!* (Hell, back when I weighed 270 lbs. I could—and often did—eat 2-3 whole packages of Reese's Peanut Butter Cups at a time, which would have been 15 servings according to the Atkins company!)

So I did the math...

18 carbohydrates x 5 servings = a staggering **90 grams of carbs** in this one small package of Atkins "diet" sweets...and this from a company that at some point in time in the past (i.e., when the pioneering Dr. Atkins was still alive) promoted a low-carbohydrate message!

The moral of the story: check the serving sizes in the products you're evaluating and do the math, if necessary.

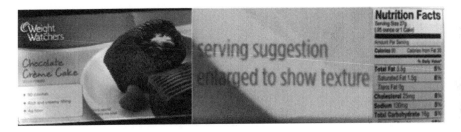

Above you'll see another example of an organization that ostensibly promotes "weight loss" but which actively markets and sells high-sugar, high-carbohydrate "food" to its customers...and then does its best to *trick* these customers into believing this krap isn't really all that bad for them.

Notice that the Nutrition Facts on the *back* of the box of Weight Watchers' Chocolate Crème Cakes clearly state that the calories and carbohydrates in the product are based on a Serving Size of 1 Cake—yet the front of the box shows *2 Cakes* and specifically notes in the text box I've enlarged for you that the picture represents the actual *Serving Suggestion*.

Why are they telling us the sugar and carb damage done by only 1 cake when they are specifically expecting us to eat at least 2 of them?!

I found some words in the thesaurus for this kind of

practice: deception, trickery, manipulation, ruse, subterfuge and dishonesty among them!

Are they trying to help people lose weight?! Or are they selling Used Cars here?! 'Cause you can't do both—you gotta pick one.

From The People Who Put the "Die" in Big Diet

Big Diet *knows* that the average overweight person eating the Krap they sell isn't going to stop and analyze the packaging long enough to realize there's a Bait & Switch going on, that the Serving Size in the Nutrition Facts on the back of the box is only half of the actual sugars and carbohydrates of the suggested serving size of 2 Cakes depicted on the front.

At 16 grams of carbs per cake, the suggested serving size of just two of these little things contains a whopping *32 grams* of carbohydrates, which means the all-too-familiar blissful Insulin-rush and attendant fat-storage is soon to follow.

Like Atkins, Weight Watchers has apparently either never heard of the advantages of a low-carb lifestyle or else they abandoned it long ago in favor of high-carb profits for the Big Food corporations who own them and whose publicly traded stocks depends on *increasing sales* rather than *decreasing waistlines*.

And even the *suggested Serving Size* for these Chocolate Crème Cakes is a little suspect, since many people would find it difficult to stop eating after merely 2 of these teensy-weensy cakes!

I mean, these little bitches are tiny, tiny, *tiny*! Back when I weighed practically 270 lbs., if I'd been presented with a box of these cakes I would have had to devour at least 4-5 of these little things to get the slightest feeling of anything in my stomach...which would've meant an overdose of 64 to 80 grams of carbohydrates to my system, and a certainty that I would remain fat for yet another day until my bloodstream could recover from the shock of this experience.

The take-away here is that if we cannot even trust organizations whose marketing is theoretically built around helping people lose weight, then we certainly cannot trust any of their fellow members of Big Food who don't even pretend to care one way or another about our health or our waistlines.

So always read the back of the box…except for food-shaped products from Big Diet, in which case you should always read the back and the front of the box, lulz!

What's The Score?

Okay, let's recap where we are…

We're *not* counting calories or weighing portions or concerning ourselves in any way, shape or form with the *amount* of food we eat. That's not really a factor in our eating decisions. We eat when we're hungry and stop when we're no longer hungry, the way all animals in the world (except goldfish, apparently!) do it.

We're avoiding excess, added sugars in our food. Sure, if you have an overwhelming craving for sweets or ice cream, go indulge that desire. But be sure to *forgive yourself* before, during and afterwards…and then return to a lifestyle where you generally avoid eating too much sugary stuff. That's a fair deal, right?!

We're avoiding wheat products because they are practically the highest scoring foods on the Glycemic Index—which is essentially a chart of how much fat any given food will store in our bodies.

As with sweets (or anything else we intend to avoid) if we do end up consuming wheat products, the best strategy is to be "okay" with it and continue moving forward with our *Low Carb Revolution* lifestyle.

We are drinking alcohol in moderation—primarily because of its hefty calorie count of 7 calories per gram which our body MUST burn off *first* before it can get back to using any energy from the foods we've eaten. In addition, alcohol summons the appetite-stimulating, abdominal-fat-creating hormone Ghrelin…while simultaneously blocking our wonderful hunger-suppressing, energy-regulating master hormone, Leptin.

And we're now also avoiding *processed* Mega-Sugars, which is to say the carbohydrates that Big Food/Big Diet deliberately stuffs into their food-shaped chemical concoctions because they *know* that carbs are both addictive and they stimulate our appetites to eat more.

> *"Low-Carb diets can today be seen as compatible with scientific evidence and best practice for weight reduction for patients with overweight or diabetes type 2, as a number of studies have shown good effect in the short term and no evidence of harm has emerged."*
> —Swedish National Board of Health & Welfare, January 2008

The Trouble With Bacon

Now don't get your panties all up in a knot at the notion that I'm about to tell you NOT to eat bacon. As with every other Progression, all I ask is that you hear me out and then make the best choice for your body. Okay, so the "trouble" with bacon is that it's a *cured* meat.

Curing is a process for preserving and flavoring meats and fish. There are all kinds of ways to cure food—using salt, smoking, using a dehydrator, etc.

The method of curing meats that Big Food prefers is

(of course!) using *sugar*. And therein lays the rub. The second or third listed ingredient (after bacon and, sometimes, water) on most commercially available packages of bacon is *sugar*.

The meat of the bacon itself scores 0 on the Glycemic Index…it's the *added sugars* that jack it up and give us that ol' familiar Insulin-Rush!

Eating bacon and other meats cured with sugars calls Insulin and leads directly to the storage of additional fat in our body.

The "low-carb" Atkins diet specifically *encourages* its followers to eat bacon, despite the fact that the sugars added to bacon in the curing process have the *exact same effect* on our bloodstreams as, say, eating a fully loaded cinnamon roll from their sister company Cinnabon—in either case the profits are flowing to the same master, the Roark Capital Group in Atlanta, GA.

But it's not all bad news about bacon. *Au contraire, Pierre!* Here's something you may not have known: we already have a perfectly healthy, non-Insulin-spiking alternative to bacon!

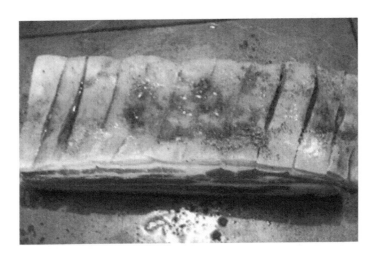

It's called Pork Belly and it's mighty fine...*might-y* fine!

The pork belly is the bottom of the big, which is exactly where commercially processed bacon comes from. And it's the most delicious thing you've probably never eaten in your life.

Pork belly is basically uncured bacon. ('Cause, you know, bacon ain't broke, so it don't need no curin'!)

The photo above shows you what a luscious slab of pork belly looks like just before I popped it in the oven. You can see the distinctive marbling of traditional bacon on the side of the cut.

But perhaps the most awesome part of pork belly is the layer of skin and fat on top. After being nicely cooked it's referred to as the "crackling"—and it's a crunchy, yumm, fatty, calorie-dense treat that, like the rest of the pork belly, scores a lucscious **0** on the Glycemic Index!

Pork belly has traditionally been considered "low rent" fare, although it's now exploding in popularity in major metropolitan areas because of its amazing taste and perfect fit into a low-carbohydrate lifestyle.

Top chefs in New York City, LA and Las Vegas have lately been crafting some spectacular dishes based around pork belly—which they refer to as the "dessert of the entrée world!"

Best of all when you're buying it at your local grocers, pork belly only costs about *half* the price of bacon!

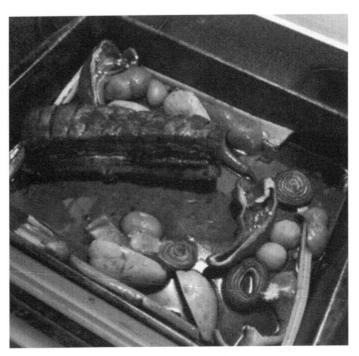

Above you can see a beautiful, fully cooked and ready-to-devour pork belly! I blasted it at 450 degrees for nearly an hour, then turned the oven down to 350 degrees for a further hour. About thirty minutes from the end of the cooking I added a few peppers, onions and veggies to give myself some variety and fiber in the meal.

So that's pork belly...and it's one alternative to traditional bacon and sausage.

Processed meats such as sausage and bacon from your local grocers are generally manufactured with excess sugars to make them more desirable to our palate and without any regard to our waistline.

In addition sausage often has wheat and soy fillers added, all of which is commonly held together with the Norman Bates of the processed food world: *Meat Glue*.

Now here's why you might want to opt for pork belly and wild-game sausage over the usual, Insulin-spiking fare: One of the most highly respected low-carb writers sometimes often gets a fair bit mean-spirited heckling on the YouTube videos of his presentations because he's, well, somewhat stocky…which would seem to belie the quite brilliant contributions he's made to the low-carbohydrate community. This (nameless, fo sho!) journalist stands 6'2" tall and *admits* to weighing 220.

He also boasts on his popular blog and virtually every interview that he devours a big ole mess o' commercially processed bacon and sausage for breakfast every morning.

I'm not sure where this otherwise *brilliant* gentleman got the idea that a morning dose of sugarized bacon and sausage was a good idea for someone advocating a low-sugar, low-carb lifestyle, but I *do* know that processed bacon and sausage has long been a mainstay of the Cinnabon, oops, I mean Atkins "diet".

In his defense, the journalist in question *is* a mesomorph.

That is to say, he possesses a naturally broad-shouldered body with big bones and plenty of muscle. Just exactly like your humble narrator, depicted below.

I'm practically a poster child for the lean, highly athletic body of a mesomorph…if not quite a poster child for modesty, lulz!

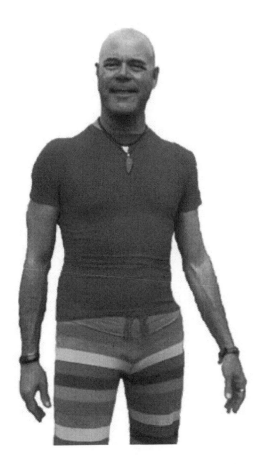

Yet despite the fact that I stand an inch taller than Mr. Bacon & Sausage Eater, I weigh only 189 lbs. — or fully 31 pounds less than he admits to.

Of course, I don't know else what this guy eats for the rest of his meals, but so far as I can tell he otherwise walks the walk of low-carbohydrate living.

The only difference between he and I besides the 31 pound differential in our weight is that he routinely starts the day with commercially processed, sugarized bacon and sausage every morning, while I "limit" myself to enjoying a huge slab of 0-GI pork belly once or twice per week.

God Is In the Details

The simple moral of the story here is to avoid excess sugars and carbohydrates in the processed, pre-made, pre-packaged foodstuffs you purchase. Look at the labels and notice what kinds of sugars and fillers that Big Food is putting into your hot dog or sausage meat.

And consider walking right past the bacon aisle and heading straight to the butcher section of your grocery store, where you can purchase mouth-watering pork belly for half the price!

Not to mention lamb and goat and other excellent meats that many people never even realize is available for the asking at your local grocers. Now that we've learned a good bit more about the processed foods we are avoiding and why, that leaves us with the very timely question of…

So What the Hell ARE We Eating?!

It's simple…we're eating *food*!

And just as much of it as we please! Personal trainer and low-carb advocate Sean Croxton teaches his clients the clever acronym, **JERF**, which stands for: **"Just Eat Real Food!"**

Here's a handy dandy chart of acceptable foods for our *Low Carb Revolution* lifestyle. We'll make a couple of *minor* tweaks to this list in the Progressions ahead, but for now all of these foods can be eaten in any combination and in UNLIMITED AMOUNTS!

LOW CARB REVOLUTION FOODS

Fruits — **All types and varieties**
Vegetables & Mushrooms — **All types and varieties**
Meat — **All types and varieties**
Poultry — **All types and varieties**
Fish — **All types and varieties**
Seeds & Nuts — **All types and varieties**

Minus the bread and modern-day Franken-wheat products, the above list essentially describes what *every human being who ever lived in the history of the world ate up until a decade or more after World War II*...real food in an infinite variety of combinations with just a small amount of added sugars.

Recall that as late as 1900, the average American ate only about 1 lb. of added sugar per year, compared to the 160 lbs. per year we were drowing in by 2010!

Food-shaped chemicals with added carbohydrates to stimulate the appetite weren't even invented until the late 1950's...so it's not like we're depriving ourselves of any actual foods here!

Bon appetit!

Progression #5: Avoid Processed Carbs
YOUR NEXT STEP...

DO avoid foods with processed sugars and carbohydrates if your goal is to let go of excess weight

DO read the labels before purchasing processed, commercially packaged meat products

DO consider treating yourself to savory pork belly rather than fat-causing, sugarized bacon

DO eat as much food as you like, whenever you like

Do NOT pay any attention to portion sizes

Special Bonus Tip: Real vs. "Pretend" Umami

Quick, what are the *four sensations of human taste*?! I'll give you 5 more seconds to think about it...4 more seconds...3...2...1!

Ha, it was a trick question!

Most of us think of the "4 basic tastes" as Sweet, Sour, Bitter and Salty.

In actual fact there's also a 5th taste, known as "umami". The term *umami* was borrowed from the

Japanese expression for a "pleasant, savory taste". Umami is that hard-to-identify quality of a food that makes it feel pleasing to our palate.

One of the reasons that ketchup is so popular is because our tongues love the umami of it. That sensation of umami perfectly blends together the sweet, the sour, the bitter and the salty of ketchup to make the sum taste even greater than the parts.

The notion of adding specific ingredients to prepared dishes to increase their umami and round out the flavors of the dish was known even by the Ancient Romans, yet it wasn't until the 20th Century that Japanese researchers discovered that amino acids known as *glutamates* were technically responsible for adding umami to dishes.

Since then, the use of glutamates to increase umami has exploded.

Glutamates are found naturally in all protein-containing foods. All meats, poultry, fish, dairy, as well as vegetables with a measure of protein, possess umami to some degree or another because of their naturally occurring glutamates—which is one reason why we enjoy eating them so much!

By the way, ALL of the naturally occurring foods in the world that contain glutamates (and which therefore possess what we could call natural umami) are on our list of *approved foods* to eat!

Big Food/Big Diet are (of course!) all too familiar with umami, and they have figured out how to synthesize glutamates in their dark, well-funded, underground laboratories and then insert them into their manufactured food products to encourage us to eat more of them.

The most popular glutamate in use today for both Asian and Western cooking is one you've probably heard a great deal about: monosodium glutamate

(MSG).

MSG is added to a tremendous number of processed foods to increase the umami. Without MSG, most low-salt or low-sugar processed foods would be so unpalatable that nobody could stomach eating more than a bite or two of them.

And even the highly processed foods that are already overflowing with salt and sugar and fillers contain plenty of umami-producing glutamates to make them more savory, more enjoyable and more addictive to customers.

These fake foods often contain little or no nutritional value, no minerals, no substance of any sort—nothing but lots of high-GI sugars and carbs to create the desired Insulin-rush in our bloodstream.

MSG By Any Other Name...

MSG itself has gotten a bad rap in recent years. I'm not going to list the growing number of health concerns about MSG other than to note that there are apparently some people who react quite poorly to it. Surprise, surprise, the commercial use of MSG has only continued to *increase*—save for the fact that Big Food/Big Diet, just like their counterparts at your local Chinese restaurant, now deliberately *disguise* their ongoing use of MSG behind other names.

A few of the common, legally "allowable" alternate names for monosodium glutamate include:

Hydrolyzed vegetable protein
In fact, anything "hydrolyzed"
Autolyzed vegetable protein
In fact, anything "autolyzed"
Yeast extract
Plant protein extract
Almost anything ending in "glutamate"

Almost anything ending in "caseinate"
Whey protein
Soy protein
Vegetable protein
Indeed, anything "...protein"
Gelatin
And the ever-popular catch all, "Natural Flavors"

Monosodium glutamate is quite purposefully placed into the fake foods we're being sold in order to artificially give them umami and thus increase our desire for them.

These food-shaped chemicals congregating in the inner aisles of our neighborhood grocery-arma are not natural foods.

Indeed, they are not "food" at all by any reasonable definition of that word. They are, quite literally, delivery systems for sugars and carbs...with enough added glutamates to make them tasty enough to swallow. Period.

Remember when you were little and you would get all annoyed when your favorite TV show was interrupted by commercials?! And then you grew up and realized the point of television *is* the commercials, because that's where the networks make all their money. The TV shows themselves exist only as a means to keep us watching until the next commercial "break".

So too, Big Food is selling us nothing more and nothing less than *the Insulin-rush from sugars and carbs.*

They only package these Insulin-spiking sugars and carbs in food-like form to give us an excuse to eat them, but they're not meant to sustain our lives, only to give us enough of an Insulin-buzz that we'll keep coming back for more!

In the final analysis, check the packaging of the foods you buy. (And remember to check both the front and the back when you're buying a food-shaped product from Big Diet!)

And when in doubt, **JERF!** Just Eat Real Food!

> *"In a time of universal deceit, telling the truth is a revolutionary act."*
> —George Orwell

PROGRESSION #6:
Avoid Drinking Sugars & Carbs

We Are What We Drink

This may be the most important progression of them all! Most of us pay little or no attention to the torrent of sugars and carbohydrates in the beverages we drink from the time we rise in the morning until the moment we retire for the night.

Yet it's been estimated that the average American consumes *20% of their total daily caloric intake in liquid form.*

We're not just eating the wrong things...we're drinking ourselves fat at an ever-increasing rate! This chapter involves some of America's favorite beverages, including sodas, fancy caffeinated concoctions and so-called "sports" drinks.

Do you recall the 160 lbs. in added sugars statistic we've already trotted out a couple times like Hester Prynne being paraded around the town square wearing her scarlet "A"?!

Have you at all wondered how it's even physically *possible* for us to eat all that much sugar (nearly ½ pound per day!) throughout an entire year?!

Well, the short answer is, we mostly don't eat it. For the most part, we are *drinking* those excess sugars!

We're drinking them in the form of sugar added to our coffee and tea. We're drinking them in the form of sugary sodas and carbohydrate-filled "sports" drinks. We're drinking them in the form of double-wide mocha-choco-latte-mamas at Starbucks. We're drinking them in super-sweetened, umbrella-topped alcoholic mixed drinks with names straight out of an Austin Powers movie.

Not only have our beverages grown sweeter and sweeter, but the sizes of them have exploded as dramatically as our pants' sizes.

Sugar, Sugar, Sugar

In 1916 Coca Cola introduced its classic "contour bottle"...a packaging concept so unique it was granted its own United States patent.

For the next 40 years— well past WWII and into the 1950's—the Coca Cola contour bottle was the de facto yardstick against which quenching one's thirst was measured. For all those years, the standard (read, only) size in which you could purchase a bottle of Coca Cola was *6.5 ounces.*

Despite its diminutive size, the 6.5 ounce bottle of Coca Cola nevertheless managed to contain some 5 heaping teaspoons of sugar, which is a pretty serious load of glucose for our bloodstream to process.

Drink one of these babies and our Insulin supply is gonna have its work cut out for it.

Even so, if we merely drank one or two 6.5 ounce bottles of Coke per week (which we did), we'd be able to limit the accumulated levels of glucose build-up to acceptable amounts. Indeed, nobody back in the '50s or '60s was getting fat off the occasional bottle of pop.

Fast forward to today, where the average American drinks *56 gallons of soda per year*—the equivalent of more than 3 bottles of the original 6.5 ounce portion of Coca Cola every single day!

That's 15+ teaspoons of sugar or, worse, sugar substitute flooding our blood supply each day— keeping our poor overworked inner Troubadour called

Insulin on the job around the clock!

And it's said that the average American teenager today consumes a staggering 800+ cans of soda per year—which doesn't even seem humanly possible until you have a teenager of your own, and then it seems like a bit of an understatement!

Size Matters

The 6.5 ounces of soda two or three times per week that our grandparents were content with seems like an almost laughably minuscule amount by today's standards.

Hell, most of us probably *spill* 6 or so ounces of soda in our haste to fill up our 44-ounce, 52-ounce and even 60-ounce cups of Coke or the like.

Now this Progression is about both our high-sugar, high-carb beverage habit and the fact that most of us barely even *notice* what we put into our bodies when it comes in the form of fluids.

One of our principal outcomes here is to become more mindful about our liquid sugars and Mega-Sugars. The sugary beverages we imbibe is the one and only area where I'm advocating anything close to portion control.

If drinking 3 soda pops per day makes us fat, then drinking a little less of it will make us a little less fat, right?! 6.5 ounces of Coca Cola a few times per week more than satisfied the thirst of two entire generations of Americans.

Then the 12 ounce can was introduced, and that quenched the thirst of two *more* generations...which neatly covers the first 80 years of Coke in America.

It's only in the most recent generation—just the past twenty years—that the sizes of our soda pops have gone through the roof. Every convenience store on every corner in America now offers soda in sizes to match our waistlines: 24 oz....32 oz...44 oz...60 oz...and more!

The growth in the sizes of our sweetened, carbonated beverages has tragically overlapped the growth of Obesity Nightmare that began in earnest back in 1992.

Our takeaway: *size matters...and, in this case, smaller is better!*

Drink Fewer Carbonated Beverages

If you intend to continue consuming soda pop — or any of the other fat-producing beverages we'll discuss — that's your personal choice.

I'd just like you to at least consider developing a new habit of drinking smaller portions of them. Even an entrenched habit of starting the day with, say, a 32 oz. cup of Dr. Pepper can evolve into a new habit of drinking "merely" a 20 oz. bottle of DP or even a 12 oz. can or, on some days, none at all.

The less we consume of sug arycarbonated beverages, obviously, the less Insulin will be called and the less fat will be produced and store in our already overburdened cells.

Using the revolutionary mind-body techniques you'll be exposed to in Part Two of the *Low Carb Revolution*, you will learn how to develop a new habit of drinking smaller portions of soda, or even none at all, if that's what you ultimately decide is best for your health and your figure.

Back when I tipped the scales at nearly 270 lbs. I drank at least two 32 oz. sodas per day.

And I paid the price for it with a bloodstream constantly awash in Insulin that dragged me down and kept me feeling listless and moody.

I virtually never drink soda anymore...although I do give myself ongoing permission to drink one should the overwhelming desire ever crop up, just as I do with all the other fat-producing substances I regularly avoid. Like Christine's cat, I like to leave the door slightly ajar, just in case!

Summing up our discussion of carbonated beverages...

Cultivate the habit of drinking smaller portions of soda. The less sucrose or artificial sweetener you introduce into your bloodstream, the less Insulin you will call and the less fat you will store and maintain. Period. Bauhaus architect Ludwig Mies van der Rohe was right all along: *less is more!*

Add a twist of lemon or lime to "de-acidify" all carbonated beverages (see the progression called "Mind your pH" for more on this topic)

Soda pop falls into the category of "lighter fluid" for the furnace of our body. It burns hot, but quickly runs out of steam, leaving us with less energy than before.

For this reason it's best not to consume it before or during any physical activity (exercising, dancing, making sweet love down by the river, etc.) because it will cause you to tire faster than otherwise.

Liquid Sugars With Caffeine

Here's a secret many people seem to be unaware of...they also sell traditional brewed coffee at Starbucks!

In fact, brewed coffee is what I always order when I go to Starbucks. Their coffee of the day is quite delightful. It also has zero carbohydrates, which means it calls zero Insulin and causes zero fat to be stored in the body. (I add a sprinkling of cinnamon to my coffee, which has long been known to stabilize blood sugars. If you choose to use an artificial sweetener, please consider using some variation of the natural sweetener, Stevia, and absolutely AVOID aspartame and its competitors.)

Good old-fashioned coffee remains one of the great delights of the world. Yet since the rise of sugary coffee-like drinks it has become almost a forgotten pleasure.

The varieties and flavors of coffee beans from around the world remain staggering in number.

I have created my very own exotic coffeehouse right in my kitchen with a simple coffee bean grinder and a French press. I have dozens of rich, flavorful packages of whole coffee beans to choose from, such that every day is a new gustatory experience. My point here, of course, is that coffee has a long, storied tradition among humans...and coffee, by itself, is a rich, tasty, highly enjoyable hot beverage.

Whereas most of the "drinks" they serve at Starbucks and the like have nothing to do with coffee as we know it.

They are essentially Liquid Sugars with Caffeine. And it will come as no surprise to you that Liquid Sugars with Caffeine overwhelm our blood supply with glucose...with the all-too-familiar result of storing still more fat in our bodies.

All of these same caveats apply to the expansive growth in super-sweetened teas, of course. Whether hot or cold, teas with added sugars and Mega-Sugars have blown up in popularity and provide undesired opportunities for us to spike our glucose and store fat without even necessarily noticing it.

My recommendations about caffeinated beverages...

Avoid Liquid Sugars with Caffeine from Starbucks-y kinds of places

If you must drink Liquid Sugars with Caffeine, cultivate the habit of ordering smaller sizes of them. (Remember the graphic earlier of Starbuck's new planned size of the "Trenta"—which contains more liquid than the human stomach is physically capable of holding!)

Explore the rich diversity of "regular" coffees. That nasty crap in the office percolator has nothing to do with the whole world of rich varieties and tasty flavors of coffee beans out there

If anything, the world of naturally caffeinated and non-caffeinated teas is even richer and more diverse than that of coffee, and many teas are dense in anti-oxidants and other beneficial micronutrients

Super-sugarized, super-carbed coffee drinks and sweetened tea drinks act like "lighter fluid" for our internal engines…burning briefly and explosively before dying out and leaving us feeling spent and out of energy

Sports Drinks Are Just "Liquid Desserts"

Sports drinks such as Gatorade, Powerade, AllSport and their ilk are downright boastful about being nothing more than chemical concoctions of sugars, carbohydrates and water.

In their multi-million dollar ad campaigns, they sell us on the "benefits" of replenishing the carbohydrates in our bodies during and after exercise—which you and I know completely and totally defeats the entire purpose of exercise in the first place.

Carbohydrates cause us to produce and maintain fat. Period.

Putting carbs into our bodies during times of exercise is like putting milk in the gas tank of our car before setting out on a road trip…just not the best idea, really!

Additionally, when we shake our booty and our heart-rate becomes elevated, an interesting physiological phenomenon takes place inside us. Our

Insulin response is *suppressed*, because our bodies want to be able to take advantage of every last drop of glucose in our bloodstreams and use if for our immediate energy needs.

This, of course, is a good thing. We *want* our Insulin to be scarce and we want our internal systems to burn the glucose already available in our blood.

In fact, we want to practically run out of glucose so that the swashbuckling hormone Glucagon will come sweeping in to the rescue and liberate stored fatty acids so we can burn those for energy as well in the process we explored earlier with the tongue-twisting name of gluconeogenesis.

The only substance we need to keep this beautiful, fat-burning factory going while we're moving our bodies is *water*...and lots of it.

Pure, unadulterated H20 is what our body craves to keep our furnace burning at max power. I can—and regularly do—dance, bike, walk, juggle, swim and play for up to 4 hours in a single day drinking water alone. I never, ever drink any sugarized, carbohydrate-laden drinks of any kind and yet I "magically" have all the energy and vitality I need to make my dreams come true each and every day.

When we exercise for twenty or thirty minutes and then pour a factory-concocted potion of sugars and carbs into our body in the form of a "sports" or "energy" drink, we immediately and dramatically spike our Insulin levels, which leads to storing the liquid dessert we just consumed directly as fat in our bodies.

Sports drinks often contain 13-19 grams of Mega-Sugars per eight ounces. The average container sizes today range from 24-32 ounces, meaning the overall carbohydrate load of that single bottle of Carb-orade is a staggering 39-76 carbs!

Hmmmmm, I wonder why Americans continue to grow more and more obese even as our gym memberships are on the rise nationwide?!

Maybe it's because we're all drinking Liquid Desserts right in the middle of our workouts and then wondering why in the world we keep gaining weight fat?! The average person doing an average (or even above average) amount of Play in a given day has no physiological need for any beverage other than water to sustain their energy levels and maintain low levels of Insulin.

On the other hand, as I've mentioned before, if you're training for an Iron Man Triathlon, different rules may apply to your training regime.

Yet for the 99.99% of humanity who will never in our entire lives need to swim for 2.5 miles and bicycle for 112 miles and run a full marathon all in a single day, then drinking sports drinks has only one benefit for us: it's the fastest way to become the fattest kid on the block!

Summing up Insulin-summoning, fat-depositing Sports & Energy Drinks...

Sports Drinks made entirely of water, sugar and carbohydrates are not only unnecessary for an ordinary active lifestyle, they are completely *counterproductive* to it

Energy Drinks made entirely of water, sugar, carbohydrates and caffeine are even *more* counterproductive to our goal of returning to our Ideal Weight

Shaking our booty creates exactly the right environment within our bloodstream of little or no Insulin and the opportunity to burn off stored fat, whereas downing a Sports or Energy Drink floods us with high Glycemic-Index carbohydrates and completely undoes every single potential benefit of our exercise session

When considering the "helpful" nutritional information about the benefits of Gatorade, for example, keep in mind they are owned by Pepsico— whose entire business model is built on the over-Insulin-ization of America.

"Sports" drinks are the ultimate "lighter fluid" fuel for our bodies. Sports drinks actively interfere with the sustained burning of the coal furnace of our cells, and instead flame out quickly on its high-GI fuel of sugars and Mega-Sugars, leaving us exhausted after a relatively modest effort compared to what we are truly capable of

"Energy" drinks are merely Sports Drinks with caffeine

Water, Water Everywhere... And Not A Drop to Drink!

Up until the 1960's most people consumed very few calories in the form of beverages other than alcoholic beverages. The vast spectrum of sugary drinks we guzzle with such regularity today literally did even exist until quite recently. Most of humanity, for most of history, drank water most of the time.

Indeed, we are the only animal on the entire planet that ever regularly drinks anything other than water in order to survive and flourish!

Carb-olicious drinks just dump more and more lighter fluid on the spreading wildfire of our global Obesity Nightmare.

Water contains no sugars, no carbohydrates and no calories. Nothing about water contributes to generating or storing fatty acids. I invite you to drink more of it. Not only does water not cause us to gain weight, it may help us to actually *lose* it.

There are some cutting-edge studies being done

right now about water and weight loss which have not yet been formally published, but the early indications are quite promising. In a nutshell, what these pioneering studies seem to show is...

People who drink more water each day regularly lose more weight regardless of their diet plan.

In other words, even if you were stuck on a worst-case scencario restricted-calorie diet where the expected total weight-loss is minimal after 12 or even 24 months of suffering, by simply increasing the amount of water these dieters drink each day they will tend to improve their results!

With a low-carbohydrate lifestyle such as we are being presented with here, drinking more water each day can only improve our already heightened expectations of excellent results.

Bottom line: *Whenever possible, drink more water!*

Progression #6: Avoid Drinking Sugars and Carbs
YOUR NEXT STEP...

DO avoid drinking beverages with excess sugars and Mega-Sugars...or at least consider consuming smaller portions

DO review the specific recommendations listed for Soda, Coffee and Sports/Evergy Drinks

DO drink more water to maximize your weight loss

DO add a twist of lime or lemon to your drinks (yes, even to your water!) whenever possible to help promote a desired alkaline pH within your body

"The miracles are within you!"
—Paul Bragg

Special Bonus Tip: Add A Twist of Lime

I've got another special bonus tip for you. This specific strategy has nothing particularly to do with weight, but much to do with our internal health!

All of the beverages we've explored in this progression of Soda Pop, Coffee and Sports/Energy Drinks have *acidic* effects on our bodies, which is not a good thing.

We'll explore the topic of our delicate internal pH balance in a future chapter, but for now let me assure you that our bodies prefer a slightly alkaline environment and will do anything (and I mean *anything!*) to preserve that.

Human pH optimally ranges from 7.35-7.45. Our internal pH is so narrowly monitored that a deviation of merely .01 is cause for serious issues within us (such as acidosis) and a deviation by .5 can kill us dead.

Beyond the effect of spiking our glucose when consumed, carbonated beverages, sugary coffee drinks and "sports" drinks add to our acidity.

So I want to share with you a little Mediterranean trick that'll help you offset the acidity of these beverages.

Although citrus fruits like lemons and limes are acidic by nature, they essentially have an alkaline effect on your body which can help counteract the acidity of these drinks. All you need to do is squeeze a twist of fresh lemon or lime into your soda or (heaven forbid you still drink them!) your sports drink.

If you dare, you can even take bites of lemon or lime to neutralize the acidic effect of your morning coffee. In Italy, the women regularly peel and eat whole limes while spending the afternoon drinking strong coffee with their friends—they instinctively figured out that the alkaline effect of limes helps restore pH balance to their bodies.

Give the lemon or lime trick a try! You may be pleasantly surprised by how much better your stomach and whole body feels when you maintain a more neutral or even slightly alkaline internal environment!

"Too much of a good thing can be wonderful."
—Mae West

PROGRESSION #7:
Avoid Natural Carbs

Nature's Carbohydrates

All plant-based foods, whether fruit or vegetable, contains some measure of carbohydrates and sugars. Most fruits and vegetables have relatively modest amounts of each, but there are a few plant foods that have either elevated carbohydrates (complex sugars) or elevated fructose (simple sugars) to such a degree that I'm going to recommend that you eat less of them.

As always, keep in mind the nature of the progressions we're making as we refine our lifestyle here. Each progression is a refinement or tweaking of the steps that went before it.

Only begin implementing a new progression—this one or any other—when you feel comfortable and confident about your own personal progress in creating new habits and lifestyles out of the ones that came before.

This particular chapter will be short and sweet...literally!

Our focus is on learning to avoid just a few particular fruits and vegetables that do no serve us when our goal is to let go of stored fat and return to our Ideal Body.

Nature's Candy Jar

Fruits are wonderful, healthy sources of all sorts of vitamins, nutrients and what are known as *phytochemicals*. Basically phytochemicals are the "tonsils" of the nutrition world. They consist of small (often minuscule) quantities of diverse nutrients that are found in all plant-based foods and whose exact purpose is often little known and/or little appreciated. Sort of like our tonsils!

Now there are some low-carb enthusiasts who go so far as to suggest we avoid or even eliminate all fruit from our diets.

There's a word for these people: curmudgeons! Besides the dozens of vitamins and minerals in fruits, they contain thousands (some would say tens of thousands) of healthy, helpful phytochemicals, which play all sorts of essential roles at a cellular level in our body.

Is it possible to overdo it on fruit?! No doubt. But the vast majority of us have the opposite problem: we eat far too little fruit rather than too much of it.

And here's the deal...

Although one of our principal goals together is certainly to lose weight, another significant objective is to restore our health.

So even if the fructose in fruit don't always mind our waistline, eating fruit does serve our overall health. I think of fruit as nature's own candy jar...and if you become a regular eater of fruit you will seldom have cravings for artificial sweets made of processed sugars.

"Fructose, a sugar from fruits, causes a significant release of Insulin only in the presence of previously elevated blood sugar."
— Morrison Bethea, MD, Sam Andrews, MD, Leighton Steward & Luis Balart, MD in *SUGAR BUSTERS!*

Eat Fruit On Its Own

The other significant thing to remember about fruit—besides eating it regularly!—is to eat it separately from vegetables and animal foods.

We digest fruit in a completely different fashion than we digest anything else. Our intestines put fruit on a fast track.

Fruit can be processed and pass through us in as little as 20 minutes...making it, by the way, the perfect source for immediate energy if you're ever out spending a whole evening dancing or somesuch! Traditional food, on the other hand, can take 2-4 hours or more to make its circuitous journey through meandering Amazon river of our small and large intestines.

Rather than risk having the fruit get caught up *behind* all that mess, it's less stressful for our bodies and less labor for our digestive systems to eat fruit all by its lonesome, then wait 20 or so minutes before digging into a meal of meat, veggies, etc.

I'll spare you any further details on the science of how we digest fruit, other than to mention that it is all quite fascinating.

If you'd like to learn more about why it's beneficial to eat fruit separately from other foods, I recommend Harvey and Marilyn Diamond's classic book, *Fit for Life*.

I also strongly advocate the book Fit for Life *if your goal is to incorporate the principles of the* Low Carb Revolution *into a vegetarian lifestyle.*

Avoid Super-Sweet Fruits

Without further ado, let's consider a few restrictions to our own personal fruit-opia.

There's a mere handful of fruits with such high

levels of sugars or Mega-Sugars that we should normally avoid eating them, and surely never over-indulge in them.

The list of super-sweet fruits to avoid is thankfully short:

Bananas
Mango
Papaya
Pineapple

Eat these (and similar island-y, tropical fruits) sparingly, if at all.

By the way, the fruits with the *lowest* concentration of sugars and carbohydrates/saccharides are the "berries". These include:

Strawberries
Blackberries
Blueberries
Huckleberries
Boysenberries
Cranberries

Eat plenty of berries…your body will love you for it!

Avoid High-Carbohydrate Cereal Grains

The next category of *natural* foods that nevertheless rank high enough on the Glycemic Index that we should avoid them are a few additional cereal grains. Wheat products are so pervasive and so harmful to our glucose levels that we covered them in their own separate progression, but there are some other grains we want to avoid because they also score so high on the GI.

We're not gonna get all nit-picky and banish every type of cereal grain known to humanity from our dinner plate. Instead we're just going to pick on two categories that are not only hugely popular but also cause us to become huge.

And these are:

Rice (white and brown)
Oats

Although brown rice does contain a marginally more fiber than white rice, it stores exactly the same amount of fat in our bodies as white rice and so should be avoided.

Both brown and white rice rank a whopping 59 on the Glycemic Index—*making rice identical to eating raw table sugar!*

A common question is: "But what about Asians—don't they eat rice all the time without becoming obese?"

The quick answer is: True dat! The traditional Asian diet was indeed high in carbohydrate-laden rice, *but* it was also super-low in all other forms of sugars and carbohydrates, and featured a diverse array of fish and seafoods.

The slightly longer answer is: If you move to Japan and join a Buddhist monastery, say, and eat their old-fashioned, traditional diet, you will do just fine. However, the Japanese population at large is now starting to experience an obesity trend of their own as they add more and more sugars and Western carbohydrates to their traditional diet.

And it's well-documented that when Asians move to the United States and combine their rice-alicious diet with the modern American High-Carb lifestyle that their obesity levels go straight through the roof just like the rest of us.

Avoid High-GI Vegetables

If you call to mind the list of high-Glycemic Index foods we've trotted out a couple of times already, you may remember that at the very top of the list—higher than any other item—was the Potato with a whopping GI of 98!

Just as there are some super-sweet fruits we should generally avoid, so too there are some super-high GI vegetables that spike our glucose and contribute to the Insulin-ization of our entire bodies.

To recap the GI scale…

At the bottom are foods that score 0 or very close to it, like most vegetables and all animal products, followed by fruits, nuts and beans a little higher up but still within our desired guidelines. Towards the middle are foods high in simple sugars, such as the super-sweet fruits we mentioned earlier, as well as any food or drink containing good, old-fashioned table sugars or some variation thereof. Near the top are foods high in Mega-Sugars, such as breads, oats, rice, grains and all foods made from wheat products.

And at the very tippy-top of the GI come the only food group that is worse for us than even wheat products, and these are the starches.

These can range from manufactured starches such as rice starch, tapioca starch and corn starch—often used in gluten-free cooking, by the way, which is why you should always run screaming in the opposite direction when offered a bite of most commercially manufactured gluten-free products!--to foods that *naturally* contain excessive amounts of starches.

And it is these latter, natural foods that contain a large amount of top-of-the-GI starches that we now turn our attention.

Like the others, this final category contains foods

that are naturally occurring but which should nevertheless be avoided.

These are the vegetables that spike our blood sugar and are more responsible for high levels of fat-depositing Insulin than just about anything else we can consume short of mainlining High Fructose Corn Syrup directly...

Potatoes
Sweet Potatoes
Beets
Carrots
Corn

In other words, many of the most popular "root vegetables."

An easy rule of thumb to gauge the starchiness of a food is to consider how difficult it is to cut while still uncooked. If you gotta whip out a damn chainsaw to cut through a raw vegetable in order to prepare it for cooking, you can pretty well guarantee it's high in starches — which are essentially mega-carbohydrates. (I guess that would make them Mega-Mega-Sugars, which sounds almost like a fictitious sorority name from the movie *Animal House!*)

As the authors of *SUGAR BUSTERS!* put it: "Potatoes, beets, carrots and many other root vegetables are simply starch, a storage form of glucose. Once inside our digestive tracts, they are quickly converted to pure sugar. Their absorption is rapid, and the resulting Insulin response is very significant."

It's worth mentioning that although corn does have a fair bit of starch in it, the real problem with corn is the inflated amount of sugars that have been deliberately bred into contemporary versions of it.

The corn that American Indians ate ranged from 1-3% sugar. In order to make corn (and all its many,

many by-products, such as corn chips, corn tortillas and the like) more attractive and addictive, over the years Big Food has quietly and deliberately altered its genetic structure to produce ever higher sugar contents.

The corn available in American grocery stores today consists of a whopping *25% sugars*...and the next generation of corn currently in development will exceed is *33% sugar*! (Big Food's entire business model behind this genetically modified, super-sweetened corn is that the sweeter it becomes, the more we will eat of it.)

Again, every foodstuff derived from corn also contains that same unhealthy percentage of sugars, which is why we're also taking pains to avoid corn chips, corn tortillas, corn flakes and on and on.

Ditto potatoes and its subsidiary products.

Indeed, potatoes have had as profound an impact on our collective Obesity Nightmare as virtually any other food, as well as its many high GI derivatives such as French fries, potato chips, hash browns, mashed potatoes, tater tots...well, I think you get the idea!

Progression #7: Avoid Natural Carbs
YOUR NEXT STEP...

DO avoid high-sugar tropical fruits such as Banana, Papaya, Mango and Pineapple

DO avoid high-carbohydrate (Mega-Sugars) cereal grains such as Rice and Oats

Do avoid high-starch (Mega-Mega-Sugars!) vegetables such as Potatoes, Corn, Carrots and Beets...and all the many snack foods made from them

SPECIAL BONUS TIP: Automate Breakfast and Lunch

I learned about "automating" meals from diet maven Jorge Cruise, who himself learned it from Dr. Mehmet Oz, so the concept has a nice little lineage behind it!

The simple, yet quite clever, idea here is to "automate" one or more of our meals per day so we don't even have to think about them and we can take the decision-making process completely out of the mix.

What I eat for breakfast fluctuates a bit over the course of the year. During the summer I eat more fruit and during the winter I eat more protein first thing in the morning. But in both cases I often start the day with fat—such as a couple of spoonsful of raw coconut oil.

Meanwhile, I've automated my lunch-making process to feature a stir-fry that I whip up at home my trusty iron skillet.

Even though I make a stir fry for lunch almost daily, it's never the same thing twice. The foundation of my stir fry is whatever veggies I have at hand.

A good rule of thumb for vegetables is to cook "across the color scale" as much as possible. In the stir fry depicted above you'll notice the red of radishes and tomatoes, green from bell peppers and jalapeños, purple from cabbage, and the like.

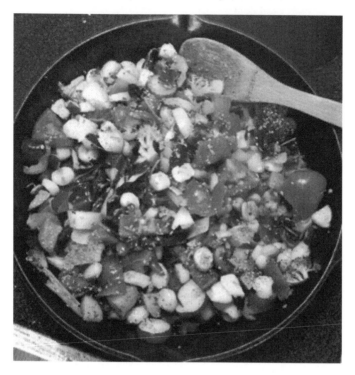

I also usually toss in some manner of protein or another: ground beef, pork, chicken or fish.

With the virtually infinite potential combination of veggies and proteins that go into my daily lunch time stir fry, the meal may well be "automated", but it's far from ever being the exact same thing twice! Also note the flax seeds sprinkled on top for extra Fiber. I commonly also add uncooked garlic, parsley and cilantro on top after the rest of the meal is complete. Many herbs (such as these three) are healthier when eaten raw or as close to raw as possible.

Years before I learned about the concept of "automating meals" I was already doing so, regularly eating fruit for breakfast and a simple veggie + protein stir fry for lunch.

When I later heard Jorge Cruise talk about it, the concept not only made perfect sense but it also put a *label* on what I'd already been doing without even knowing why!

Taking away our ad hoc decision-making process for one or even two meals per day by automating them means we're much more likely to eat foods that serve us and serve our goal of releasing belly fat than if we woke up each day and had to solve the problem of what we were going to eat for every single meal that day from scratch.

And the result of automating or semi-automating (as with breakfast) my first two meals of the day is that my dinner can be, well...anything.

Dinner is the meal where I throw routine out of the window and decide to go out to eat or decide to grill a whole fish on banana leaves on the barbeque grill or decide to munch on a raw feast of avocados, mushrooms, nuts and olives...or whatever else I may desire that contains some combination of protein, fat and fiber—and with no excess or added carbohydrates, to be sure!

"There is a real magic in enthusiasm. It spells the difference between mediocrity and accomplishment."
—Norman Vincent Peale

PROGRESSION #8:
Mind your pH

Test the Water Before You Jump In

If you've spent much time around swimming pools then you know that checking the pH level of the water is an essential aspect of keeping it fit for human use.

Much like pools, our bodies consist largely of water, which also must be maintained at a very precise pH level.

The pH scale reflects a balance between acidity and alkalinity. The scale goes from 0 – 14, with 0 being the most acidic and 14 being the most alkaline.

People fall just slightly north (towards alkaline) of the center of the scale. The human body is a tightly controlled pH vessel. Deviate up or down by merely half a point from our normal pH of around 7.4 and we will die.

Our beautiful bodies prefer a slightly alkaline environment. Unfortunately most of the vices of the modern-day world are highly acidic.

As our pH level drops because of the accumulated acidity, our body becomes weaker, more fatigued and less able to function at anything approximating normal levels.

When our bodies are in an acid state, there's a certain amount of continual internal corrosion going on that's a lot like that nasty-ass rust that can build up on the battery terminals in the car.

This acidic corrosion within us may go unnoticed

for years, yet it keep slowing us down and shorting out our micro-circuits. As the acidity builds up in our body over time, our oxygen levels eventually begin to decline—creating a Perfect Storm where cancer cells flourish. Unlike our normal, healthy cells which prefer alkaline, oxygen-rich environments, cancer cells love the acidic, low-oxygen surroundings that are unfortunately the natural byproduct of our high-carbohydrate, high-acid lifestyles.

> *"We have become too full of acid and as a result are experiencing a wide range of diseases that flourish in the acid medium."*
> —Dr. Mary Ruth Swope

It's an Acid World Out There

Where does all this acid come from? Well, from the stuff we put in our bodies, to be sure.

As we noted in the earlier progression on drinking too many Mega-Sugars, beverages such as soda pop, coffee and sugarized "sports" and "energy" drinks all increase the acidity of our bodies.

Carbonated beverages contain carbonic acid and some of them, like Coca Cola, also contain phosphoric acid. The extreme acid loads of these carbonated sodas stretch our body's acid-neutralizing capacity to its limits.

Apart from the fat-storing repercussions of sucrose in regular sodas and neuron-damaging artificial sweeteners in diet ones, the *acidity* of the drinks themselves create a devastating effect on our pH. Carbonated beverages have a shockingly low acidity of 2...which is just slightly higher than the surface of Venus! Gatorade is not much better with a pH of 3 and even our old pal coffee weighs in at a grim 4.

The low numbers of these drinks sends our teeth

into what is referred to as "acid shock", which eats away at our enamel.

And you can only imagine what all that acid does as it descends into the soft tissues of our body. Remember the movie *Alien* where the creature's acid-blood burned through the steel decks of the commercial towing spaceship Nostromo like salt on a slug?! That's not far off from what *acid* we drink is doing to the inside of us.

Common symptoms of an unbalanced, overly acidic pH include: heartburn, bloating and belching...as well as insomnia, water retention, migraines and fatigues.

Maybe you know people who sometimes suffer from these annoying symptoms of an overly acidic lifestyle?! Maybe you know them, as Tony Robbins likes to say, *intimately*...because they are you?!

Another major producer of acid within our bodies comes from smoking tobacco...or smoking anything, for that matter.

Over time, all this acid within us takes its toll. And it's a heavy toll, indeed.

Acidity and Loss of Bone Density

It's not just our vices that contribute to our high levels of acidity. Although eating animal proteins such as beef, chicken, lamb, fish and so on are a mainstay of human life, we also get acids from their meat. Indeed all animal products—including milk, dairy and eggs—have an acid effect on body, although in their defense they do also seem to have at least some built-in mechanisms for reducing the very acid load they cause.

It's easy to ignore all this. It's downright tempting to believe that we can continue to eat and drink virtually anything we desire and just take a Tums or something to balance it all out.

While a Tums or three may well help our immediate heartburn, it does not, of course, address the desperate negotiations going on deep within our bodies because of the relentless acidic danger zone we've plunged it into.

Acids drive down our pH, which triggers a panic response from our body to compensate. (Never lose sight of the rather significant point that if our normal pH of 7.35 – 7.45 drops so much as half a point to 6.85, for example, the result will be *death*.)

Our body is therefore forced to sacrifice our long-term quality of life in order to stay alive from moment to moment.

The body does this by drawing from any alkaline store available, including the calcium phosphate in the very bones of our skeleton. Because maintaining a normal pH is so crucial to our survival, our body will sacrifice bone health to keep that pH stable level.

This is a primary reason behind the explosion of osteoporosis we're now experiencing. Our body will literally turn our entire skeletal system to *mush* before its internal pH level is allowed to veer off course enough to threaten our life as a whole.

Fortunately we have a ready supply of calcium carbonate and calcium phosphate in our bones to maintain the body's preferred pH of around 7.4. Unfortunately, this leeching of alkaline material causes bone loss and decreases our bone density.

Because of our highly acidic lifestyle, we regularly force our body into a Sophie's Choice of destroying our own bones from the inside-out to keep the rest of us alive.

After years of living an overly acidic lifestyle, including a staggering 4-5 pack a day cigarette habit (sic!), in 2010 I had to have each of my hips replaced in separate operations.

These full hip replacements were necessary because there literally wasn't enough bone density left in my hips to allow me to support my own weight or to walk unassisted!

You want to know a dire statistic about what happens when we don't "mind our pH"?! At age 50, more than half of American women can expect a fracture in their future!

OUCH!

You don't want that—so stay with me as we investigate ways to turn this around and finally start reducing the acidity of our magnificent bodies.

"Taking calcium supplements is no more effective at reversing bone loss than randomly tossing some bags of cement and bricks into your backyard is at building a patio."
—William Davis, MD

"One May Smile and Smile, Yet Be a Villain"

The above quote from Billy Shakespeare speaks volumes to the entire issue of acidity within us. Just because a food seems *benign* or non-acidic, doesn't make it so. (And the opposite is also true!)

Bread, for example, would appear to be alkaline. After all, it doesn't look, smell or taste remotely acidic. In point of fact, though, just as bread and wheat products rank at the very top of the Glycemic Index, they also generate more acidic byproducts than virtually any other foods. Wheat and oats are potent delivery systems of bone-devouring sulfuric acid.

As Dr. William Davis writes in his New York Times bestselling book, *Wheat Belly*, "Grains such as wheat account for 38 percent of the average American's acid load, more than enough to tip the balance into the acid range. Wheat shifts a diet that had hopes of being net alkaline to net acid, causing a constant draw of calcium out of the bones."

On the flip side, certain foods with an acidic

appearance can in reality become our #1 allies in restoring and maintaining equilibrium within our internal pH balance, and we're going to become acquainted with a couple of these.

Vegetables and fruits are the finest and foremost sources of alkalinity available to us.

As a general rule, almost everything in the produce department of your local grocery store drives our pH in the desired alkaline direction. Generous consumption of fruits and vegetables helps neutralize the acidic burden from animal products, coffee, sodas, alcohol, smoking and the like.

Here's another secret of weight loss to integrate into your life…

Losing weight isn't just about dropping pounds…it's also about restoring balance and harmony in our body!

If our journey were only to make the numbers on the scale descend as rapidly as possible until we reached our Ideal Body, then the optimum food to eat all day every day would of course be Pemmican—the concentrated, nutritious staple of animal protein and animal fat invented by Native Americans.

Because both protein and fat score 0 on the GI scale, it's basically impossible to create or store fat while living on Pemmican alone.

However, we wouldn't have a great quality of life if Pemmican was truly all we ate. Beyond protein, fat and fiber, we also require regular doses of essential vitamins, minerals and phytonutrients to flourish, all of which we get from plant foods.

As Robert Lustig, MD is fond of saying, "When nature makes the poison, it often packages it with the antidote."

Balancing our protein and fat consumption with

fresh fruits and vegetables creates a more harmonious (and *hormone*-ious!) environment in our bodies — thus preserving our internal balance and maintaining our bone density so we can remain physically active and robust throughout our entire lives, rather than hobble painfully through what are supposed to be our golden years.

As mentioned earlier, citrus fruits such as lemons and limes are especially beneficial to us. While seemingly acidic in nature, lemons and limes have a highly alkaline impact on our body.

Because of their desirable alkaline influence on our internal systems, lemons and limes should be used frequently in our cooking and also squeezed into alcoholic or carbonated beverages whenever possible to neutralize the acidic effects.

Progression #8: Mind Your pH
YOUR NEXT STEP...

DO continue to avoid highly acidic drinks such as carbonated beverages and so-called "sports" drinks

DO continue to avoid wheat products, which create enormous acid loads in our internal systems

DO be mindful that coffee, alcohol and smoking (anything!) are all highly acidic to our bodies

DO eat leafy green vegetables — as well as a broad mixture of vegetables and fruits — on a regular basis to help balance out your pH levels

DO add a squeeze of lemon or lime directly to foods and drinks whenever possible to help promote a healthy, alkaline environment

"The higher your energy level, the more efficient your body. The more efficient your body, the better you feel and the more you will use your talent to produce outstanding results."
— Tony Robbins

PROGRESSION #9:
Mix It Up!

Our Internal Efficiency Experts

The human mind is incredibly efficient at learning new processes and adopting new habits.

In truth, the mind likes to learn things as quickly as possible and store these new learnings in our body as habits less for reasons of *efficiency* than out of pure, unadulterated *laziness*.

Our brain is inherently lazy and the less time it has to spend "thinking about the same old shit", the happier it seems to be.

That's why our mind prefers to learn new things so well that it no longer has to ever think about them anymore.

Once our mind learns the directions to our new office building or how to count to ten in Japanese, for example, it stores that information in the "hard drive" of our *body* and then gets back to daydreaming and telling itself stories and the like.

It should come as no surprise that our physical body does exactly the same thing.

Our body is equally efficient (that is to say, lazy!) at learning new tasks, and equally masterful at streamlining them so it can eventually do these tasks with the absolute least amount of effort.

Let's say you just bought a bicycle and decide you're going to ride it to work, a journey of 5 miles. Now let's say the very first time you make that trip it strains your muscles and seems like quite an arduous expenditure of energy, and the trip to work takes a total of, let's make up a number, say, *100 Exercise Units*.

After you've ridden to work (and, presumably, back

home again!) a bunch of times, however, the muscles in your body in charge of pedaling your bicycle become more and more efficient at doing their job.

In this manner, after just a few weeks on your bike it might take you only 65 Exercise Units to make the trip. And after a few months of riding the same route five times per week it might finally only take you *38 Exercise Units*.

Your bicycle commute hasn't changed at all. The distance remains the same. The hills remain the same. The only thing that's changed is the energy your muscles expend to make the trip—which goes *down* steadily the more you repeat exactly the same activity.

When my fellow Austinite Lance Armstrong was in mid-career, his *off-season* training rides lasted 6-7 straight hours or more. Anything less simply wouldn't been much of a strain on his ultra-efficient leg muscles.

If our goal is to create harmony and balance in our minds, our bodies and our life as a whole, then naturally we don't want to become too efficient at any of our regular activities. Is this making sense?!

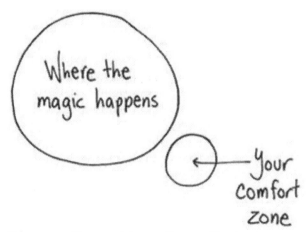

It's worth making the effort to continuously challenge our minds, bodies and limitations by pushing and changing and redefining our comfort zones as often as possible.

In other words, the more we *mix it up*, the more we'll be challenged.

And the more we're challenged, the smarter we become, the lighter we become, the faster we become and the funnier we become. (It's all true, even the funny part...stick with me on this!)

Animals Don't Move in A "Straight Line"

No animals in the world other than humans move in a straight line...or even in a circle, for that matter. We are the only animals who deliberately choose to run at a steady pace for an extended period of time even when we're not being actively chased by something that could eat us.

The only other animals who do similar repetitive movements over and over and over again like humans are zoo animals in the midst of a nervous breakdown.

All creatures in the wild move in fits and starts. Imagine that you own a dog and you let her out in the backyard. What's the first thing she does? Most likely she bolts out the door like she was shot out of a cannon—and careens directly towards the back fence, and then skids to a halt. Then she just stands there for a long moment. In the next instant, she's racing around the perimeter. Moments later, she stops in her tracks to make pee pee. Shortly after that, she's trying to climb a tree to reach a squirrel. And then she lays down in the grass, checks out completely, and takes a nice little nap. And then she's up and running again. Nothing about what she does has anything to do with moving continuously in straight lines or circles.

The natural world doesn't just ebb and it doesn't just flow...it takes turn doing each.

Sometimes creatures in the wild walk at a steady

gait to get somewhere, but along the way they sometimes sprint, sometimes sleep, sometimes stop to graze and sometimes stand around listlessly for lack of food.

The stop-start, fast-slow, herky-jerky lifestyle of the animal kingdom is actually far more enlivening and invigorating to our body (and our mind) than the traditional birth-til-death Bataan Death March of grim, constant productivity that most industrialized humans sign up for.

Another little-known secret to losing weight and keeping it off...

The secret to losing weight is to keep your body guessing about what's about to happen next!

The P90X Example

P90X is a DVD-based exercise program sold primarily via half-hour infomercials on television. It's a high-energy, high-intensity training regimen that can turn ordinary people into absolutely ripped physical specimens.

Now I've never done P90X personally because I don't believe in exercise—more on this later—but I do highly admire the *theory* behind their workouts.

The creators of P90X also understand that no animals move in straight lines. Creatures in the natural world sprint, stop, walk, eat, sprint, jump and just constantly "mix it up".

As a result, no animals of any kind—beast, fish or fowl—in the wild are overweight, much less obese. And their bodies never know what to expect next, because the animals themselves never know what to expect next.

The beauty behind the P90X program is that it duplicates the always-changing algorithm of the natural world.

And they accomplish this by requiring you to execute a completely different type of workout each week or so. One week you're doing strength training. The next week, cardio. The next week, isometric exercises. Each and every week for 6 or 9 weeks or however long the thing is you're doing something different. Always changing body movements. Always mixing it up.

As a result, your body never figures out the pattern and, most importantly, it never learns how to become overly efficient (i.e., lazy) at doing any particular activity.

So your body keeps extracting the highest possible number of my pretend unit of measure, the so-called Exercise Units, from your activities and as a result your training turns you into a lean, mean, fighting machine!

Play Like An Animal

Now I don't personally believe in lifting weights or going to a gym or doing any kind of repetitive exercise. I believe in Play.

For me, play can mean any one of dozens of physical activities…and I regularly rotate through them during the course of the year to keep my body guessing about what it's supposed to do next.

In the summertime I swim daily. In the wintertime, I hardly ever swim. In the summertime, I spend upwards of 2 hours a day rolling around town on my bicycle. In the wintertime I'm lucky to get on my bike for an hour per week. Sometimes I juggle more than at other times. Sometimes I walk more. And almost daily, year round, I dance.

But even there I'm doing different styles of dancing all the time. The broad rule behind my theory of exercise is to mix it up and keep things a little chaotic, so my body cannot predict what it will be expected to do in the future.

As a result, I have the fit, muscular body of a triathlete without the inconvenience of doing all the many hours of daily arduous exercise that actual triathletes are required to do!

And I recommend the same course of activity to you. When it comes to your "exercise program" then, don't exercise...and don't have a program! Instead of exercise, *play!* And instead of a regular schedule of play...do things slightly different each day, each week, each month, etc.

The more you mix it up and the less your body knows what's coming next, the leaner and fitter you can become with far less expenditure of energy than traditional runners and such with their habitual, joint-grinding, body-numbing workouts.

Try new things, learn new physical skills. If you don't know how to salsa dance, take lessons and go do that for a while...and then *don't* do that for a while as you do something different!

In the end, our goal is nothing short of complete and utter chaos for the body.

You want your body to constantly be trying to keep up with you and figure out what you want from it. And if it never catches up, then it also never gets a chance to get too lazy or fall into a rut.

Oh, and guess who loves, loves, loves playing this game?! Your BODY, that's who!

When you start really using your body...and not just using it, but *confusing* it, well then your body wakes up and comes alive like never before.

It's no different than waking up a puppy from a long nap. Once it's awake, it is ready to play!

> *"Play is the only way the highest*
> *intelligence of mankind can unfold."*
> —Joseph Campbell

Mix It Up When You Eat

I eat well virtually every single day. But I do not eat well in the exact same *way* every single day.

Although I generally automate my first two meals, I quite frequently throw that automation out the window and do something different.

One day I'll eat pretty much only meat from morn til night. The next day I might eat mostly raw vegetables. For the whole next week I'll go back to my automated pattern of eating, and then suddenly go on a kick of eating fish everyday for lunch for the next while. And then, to really mix things up, on other days I'll skip one, two or even all three meals just to keep my body guessing.

No two days of eating are the same...and no week is the same as the week before or the week to come...unless it just happens to turn out that way, of course!

Just as I don't want my body to know the method behind my madness of playing, I also don't want my stomach to know what's coming next in the cooking department.

Some days I'll eat only fruit every day for breakfast. Except when I don't. Usually I follow the best practice of eating 30-50 grams of protein within half an hour of waking up. Except for those days when I don't eat anything for breakfast at all. The big takeaway here is that we all operate at our best when we're kept a little bit on our toes and remain awake and alert to whatever's about to happen next.

In his popular book *The 4-Hour Body*, gadfly Timothy Ferriss champions taking off an entire day

277

each week from a sensible eating regime. He calls it a Break Day, and on that day he reommends going out of your way to eat as much Krap as you can stand eating.

I heartily endorse the concept — although I feel that if you're gonna load up on sugars and seriously harmful foods that a Break *Meal* is a better option than a whole day of it.

And, of course, the most important distinction is to mix up the day that you take your Break Day (or Break Meal), so that you do it on Saturday one week, and then skip the next week, and then do it on Wednesday at lunch and so on!

Our minds, our bodies and every aspect of our lives benefit from mixing it up and moving through the world without too much predictability. Every part of you, inside and out, appreciates variety...so indulge yourself!

> *"The only people for me are the mad ones, the ones who are mad to live, mad to talk, mad to be saved, desirous of everything at the same time, the ones who never yawn or say a commonplace thing, but burn, burn, burn, like fabulous yellow Roman candles exploding like spiders across the stars."*
> —Jack Kerouac

The More We Play, The Better We Feel

Playfulness isn't just a state of mind. It's also a state of body. And play shouldn't be restricted merely to playing or even eating.

The more we introduce the spirit and practice of play into other arenas of our life, the more youthful and energetic and curious about the world we become. Every facet of our being — body, mind and spirit — loves playing, loves games and loves surprises.

278

Here's yet another closely guarded secret about losing weight...

Losing weight isn't about a steady, daily slog towards fewer and fewer pounds...it's about continuously surprising our body with unique, playful ways to eat, move and love so that the pounds drop off not as single spies, but in battalions!

You want to look younger? Act younger! Play more. Color outside the lines, in every aspect of your life. Discover different driving routes to get yourself to work, church, the grocery store.

For that matter, try a different job, a different church, a grocery store in another part of town. Try reading a completely different genre of fiction (or even non-fiction) for a change.

Get crazy...do things you typically never do, like taking a yoga class, or become a boss at hula hoop! Learn Italian or American Sign Language or the mandolin.

Take an Improvisational Comedy class...because you really ARE funnier than most people give you credit for! Our body and mind view all of these undertakings as new games to play—games that give them something unique and entertaining to do.

Seriously, I'm here to tell you that the point of losing weight isn't to weigh less. It's to give us the opportunities to PLAY more!

Progression #9: Mix It Up
YOUR NEXT STEP...

DO mix it up and keep every system of your body just a little bit curious about what's coming up next

DON'T allow yourself to fall into a routine or a rut in any area of your life—especially when it comes to how you move your body and what you put into it

The Low Carb Revolution by John McLean

Do *Play* more!

> *"The opposite of play is not work, it's depression."*
> — Brian Sutton-Smith

PROGRESSION #10:
Cook It Yourself

Play With Your Food!

Our lives are greatly improved by introducing variety whenever and wherever we can...and by doing it as playfully as possible.

Besides "mixing it up" and continually surprising your body with new foods and new ways of moving through the world, I want to invite you to develop a sense of playfulness about getting your hands messy with the selection and preparation of the food itself.

I'm talking about learning to enjoy *shopping* for food, learning to enjoy *cooking* food and learning to appreciate the entire *eating experience* more than ever before.

At the heart of what we're accomplishing together in the *Low Carb Revolution* is the deliberate rebuilding of our relationship between our bodies and the food we put in it.

For years and years that relationship was so dysfunctional that what we often ate—whether some 99¢ Krap from the McTacoHut or the $8.99 Bottomless Bowl o' Carbs at the TGIChiliGarden—had absolutely no resemblance to food as most of humanity has known it for most of history.

The way so many of us feed our magnificent bodies has more in common with ducking into a low-rent whorehouse on the wrong side of town to satisfy our cravings for love and connection than with the profoundly tactile and rewarding experience that

281

preparing and eating actual food can be.

The processed, colorfully packaged products in the center aisles of the grocery store consist entirely of a carefully concocted assemblage of high-sugar, high-carb food-shaped chemicals that keep us mired in our Obesity Nightmare.

Despite what Mrs. Dinnsdale told you in 3rd grade, I'm encouraging you to play with your food.

Playing with your food means spending time browsing the outer perimeter of the grocery store, considering all the bountiful food choices available to us...the meats, the fish, the vegetables, the fruits, the dairy and cheeses, the seeds and nuts, the olives and other actual foods.

Even the most modest neighborhood grocery store today contains a broader and deeper collection of foodstuffs (some 50,000 unique items, on average) in one place than most of our ancestors ever beheld in their whole lives!

Playing with your food entails picking it up and handling it and putting in a basket and buying it for yourself. Playing with your food involves cooking your food.

Nothing gives you more ownership and pride over the 65 trillion amazing cells of your body than preparing a meal for them.

Slow Down And Cook

For most of my adult life I never cooked so much as a single dish. Even to this day my cooking skills are rather modest, and I rely heavily on the easiest to prepare of all meals: the Stir Fry.

I own a generous-sized cast iron skillet. Almost daily I heat that sucker up on the stove. Once it gets hot, I add either olive oil or butter or coconut oil. (Bonus Tip: Waiting until the pan gets hot *before* you add the oil is the secret to keeping food from sticking to it during cooking!)

Then I start chopping up veggies—a slightly different mix each day, of course—and tossing them into the skillet.

Finally I add some source of protein: beef, pork, chicken, fish or eggs. You might ask: "But doesn't buying my own food and cooking my own food take *time* away from other stuff I could be doing?!"

You betcha! And that's the whole *point* of it!

As counterintuitive as it may seem, the more time we spend using our Body (by dancing, playing, cooking, etc.) the more productivity we get from our Minds and the healthier we get in our Bodies and the more flowing and in alignment we become in our Energies.

The secret behind my ability to write a 460-page, 115,000-word book from scratch in 7 weeks, without so much as an outline or a scrap of notes on Day 1, was the fact that every single day during that time I spent only 4 or 5 hours actually working on the *Low Carb Revolution* and another 3 to 5 hours (or more!) per day of shopping, cooking, eating and playing.

Here's a truth that goes directly against the Protestant Work Ethic hammered into us from the womb onwards...*the harder we play, the more we can accomplish.*

When You Chop Vegetables, Just Chop Vegetables

For me, dancing is playing and swimming is playing...but roaming the aisles at the grocery store deciding what to buy is also playing, and cooking is playing, and chopping the vegetables is playing.

And when we play, we are *present*. We are here. We are grounded and focused and more awake. When I'm chopping the vegetables, that's all I'm doing, I'm chopping the vegetables.

It's a quiet, simple, Zen practice, if you will. I'm not thinking about my book or the webinar I'm creating or the hot date I have lined up for Friday night. I'm not thinking about anything at all. I'm just chopping the vegetables—and, in that moment, there's absolutely no better use of my time! Neither am I listening to the radio or an audio book or the television. Those are all distractions for my Mind that take me out of the present moment and away from whatever I am doing right now.

When we're chopping the vegetables, there's no more important thing in the world for us to be doing than chopping the vegetables. If we get that part right, believe me, every other part of our lives can fall into place.

Reconnecting our Body with our Mind isn't just an essential step in the journey towards returning to our Ideal Body. In a very real sense, it is the *entire journey!*

The average American spends just a few minutes per day on food preparation...which often involves simply microwaving a highly processed, pre-cooked meal of sugars, carbohydrates and glutamates shaped and colorized to resemble something remotely food-like.

And then they sit down in front of the television and turn on the Food Network, where they watch hour-long shows about *other* people cooking and eating food.

I call this food porno—and increasingly it's taking the place of us having to actually interact with food ourselves. Food porno encourages us to sit there without moving and watch others get to enjoy cooking and eating food in all its exquisite varieties!

Besides putting us back in touch with our bodies and increasing our overall productivity in the world, there's another significant benefit to cooking our own food that is of great interest.

There is a direct correlation between letting other people cook for us and the deepening of our ongoing Obesity Nightmare.

Cooking: The Most Ancient Art

Cooking connects us with our past. Evolutionary biologists now believe that the human tradition of cooking food dates back far longer than previously imagined. Recent discoveries have shown that early man, including both *Homo erectus* and Neanderthals, were preparing meals over fire as far back as 1.9 million years ago!

Cooking with fire allowed early humans to consume enough calories and nutrition to go about the business of evolving—or whatever it is they did all day long!—in just a fraction of the time of our primate counterparts.

Homo erectus and Neanderthals (and then, about 200,000 years ago, *Homo sapiens*) spent around two hours per day cooking and consuming food.

Compared to chimpanzees, who spend up to half their waking hours feeding, we've got it good, right?!

The Less We Cook, The More We Eat

Slow Food activist, writer, filmmaker and all-around good guy Michael Polan reports that a 2003 study by a group of Harvard economists headed by David Culter found that the rise of food preparation outside the home could explain most of the increase of obesity in America.

As Polan writes, "Cutler and his colleagues found that when we don't have to cook meals, we eat more of them. As the amount of time Americans spend cooking has dropped by about half, the number of meals Americans eat in a day has climbed."

This just makes sense. Creating a meal of home-cooked hamburgers and onion rings, for example, requires a flurry of preparation and activities to pull the whole thing off.

On the other hand, we can whip through the 99¢ drive-thru window and grab a ready-made burger and an order of flash-frozen, pre-cooked onion ring-shaped chemicals within a matter of minutes.

The fact that it takes so *little* investment of our time and money to gratify a craving for Fat Foods that are guaranteed to spike our Insulin levels and contribute to the storage of additional visceral fat in our mid-section is one of the key reasons we tend to overindulge in these culinary abominations.

Say what you will about the many drawbacks and disadvantages of becoming overweight...at the very least it's sure as hell is convenient!

In his excellent, slim book, *Food Rules*, Michael Polan offers a number of "grandmother-tested" rules to shape improved eating habits in our lives. These include such gems as, "Never buy a packaged food with more than 5 ingredients" and "Don't buy your food at the same place you buy your gas."

Directly to the point of our current conversation is his food rule: "Eat all the junk food you want...that you cook yourself."

This means if you want onion rings, then you're going to have to go buy some onions and then slice up the onions and then prepare them for frying and so on.

As a result of all this effort, you're not liable to actually indulge in onion rings more than once or twice a month — if that often!

The More We Cook, The Less We Weigh

Ready for the Big Finish?! In the 2003 study of cooking patterns across several cultures referred to above,

David Cutler and his fellow Harvard economists found that obesity rates are inversely correlated with the amount of time spent on food preparation.

In other words...the more time people devote to food preparation at home, the lower their rate of obesity. Wow!

The more we cook for ourselves, the less we tend to weigh.

This is a pretty amazing and eye-opening observation!

As Michael Polan sums it up, "So cooking matters — a lot. Which when you think about it should come as no surprise. When we let corporations do the cooking, they're bound to go heavy on sugar, fat and salt. The time and work involved in cooking, as well as the delay in gratification built into the process, serve as an important check on our appetite."

It takes *time* to slow down and shop and "chop the vegetables" and cook your own food.

But, again (and again!) that is the point of it! Gaining weight is fast, easy and convenient. We can do it on the cheap and without hardly thinking about it.

Letting go of fat takes time. But time is what we have plenty of. And the more time we take in preparing our own food, the more time we actually create to let our light shine in other important areas of our lives.

If out of this entire book, the only changes you made in your life were to cut way back on the sugars and the carbohydrates in the foods you eat, along with eliminating wheat products almost entirely, and then to cook real food yourself on a regular basis, then your journey back to your Ideal Body will be a memorable and successful one.

Progression #10: Cook It Yourself
YOUR NEXT STEP...

DO prepare and cook your own food as often as possible—both to control the ingredients in it and to help reconnect with your Body

DO keep in mind the studies showing that the more we cook, the less we tend to weigh

DON'T try to simultaneously entertain your Mind while you are cooking by listening to audio/visual entertainment...cooking is about spending time with your Body

"The creation of something new is not accomplished by the intellect, but by the play instinct."
—Carl Jung

PROGRESSION #11:
Love

Love Your Tribe

Whenever we make dramatic changes in our weight or financial fortunes or other areas of life, there's often a natural temptation to want other members of our Tribe to enjoy meaningful breakthroughs of their own. Except the reality is that people change when they're ready to change and not beforehand, in exactly the same way snakes shed their skins.

For years herpetologists have tried to discern a repeatable pattern about when snakes will shed their skin—in the same way that chickens molt every fall and dogs shed regularly twice per year. but they've never been able to discover a method to the snakes' madness.

Not age, not weather, not gender—nothing in the snakes' genetics or environment gives us any clues about when they'll shed their skin or when they won't.

Finally researchers settled on the most obvious answer: Snakes shed their skins when they feel like it, period. Just like humans, who change whenever they're damn good and ready—and not a minute sooner!

So the best way to encourage other members of our Tribe to improve their own lives is to *inspire* them through our own good example.

As your friends start to notice the pounds you've lost and the glow of your healthy skin and the light in your eyes, believe me they'll take you aside and ask your secret! They're gonna want what you have: the energy, the vitality and the progress back towards your Ideal Body.

But until that moment, until they specifically request your advice on making changes in their own life, the best way to support other members of your Tribe is simply to love them.

Love them unconditionally...just the way they are right now.

If they decide to let go of carbohydrates and let go of their excess weight and begin the beautiful process of waking up, then support them unequivocally. But a certain percentage of your Tribe will never reach that tipping point in their life.

And that's okay. That's their journey through this life-cycle. Your only job is to love them and support them and be there for them just the way they are right now!

Love Yourself

A Course in Miracles teaches us that there are only two primary emotions: Fear and Love.

Eventually we let go of some of the fear and then we let go of more of the fear and still more...until ultimately all that remains is love.

At that point we realize the fear was never even there. The fear was never real, it was just something we hallucinated all along.

Finally we reach a point in our journey where love is all there is, where love is all we have and all we need. Love for ourselves, most of all. That's where the love starts, always, with ourselves.

The underlying message of every page of the *Low Carb Revolution* is to love yourself, to treat yourself as the most amazing, beautiful and unique creation in history...which is indeed the case!

One of the most tangible ways to demonstrate our

own love to ourselves is through treating our beautiful body with tender loving care. If you didn't already do the loving exercises from the Appreciate Your Body Day back in Key #4, now would be a very good time to do them. In fact, any day is a good time to appreciate and love your body!

> *"What is not Love is always*
> *fear, and nothing else."*
> — A Course in Miracles

Love Your Stomach

Most of us spend every penny of our discretionary income on informing and/or entertaining our Minds by buying every conceivable manner of books, magazines, movies, music, HD TV, etc., to keep it occupied. Yet we *skimp* when it comes to spending money on our bodies.

Sure, I am talking about springing for massages or alternative healing sessions or yoga classes and the like, each of which send a powerful message to our bodies that says, "I care about you!"

But I'm *also* talking about spending money on our stomachs and showing it some love. For over a decade of my life I was stuck on the 99¢ Hamster Wheel of Krap at McTacoHut. When I ultimately made the decision to return to my natural state and birthright of my Ideal Weight, that meant investing in actual food for myself to eat rather than the pennies-on-the-pound food-shaped chemicals I'd numbed myself to subsist on.

And real food costs money. But here's the deal…it's not that real food costs *too much* money, it's that subsisting off the dollar menu costs *too little*.

As recently as the 1980s — you know, back when most everybody was slim and the obesity level was at a reasonable 2.5% — Americans spent anywhere from 15-

25% of their income on food.

By 2010 Americans spent a miserly 9% on food and Europeans not much more than that.

One of the reasons we're in the midst of our present Obesity Nightmare is that we've been spending too little on our food.

Sugar and carbs cost next to nothing. That's why Big Food is feeding them to us. Yet the less we spend on our food, the bigger we become. You wanna show some love to your stomach and your waistline? Then spend a little money on real food for your body rather than giving every dime you earn to the service of your mind.

I know business people will spend $2000 on a ticket to a self-improvement seminar or conference, then buy airline tickets to fly halfway across the country for it and shack up in a $240 a night hotel for days on end, yet they go out of their way to subsist largely on the Bagels & Krap served by the conference hosts because it's FREE!!!

When I suggest dropping a couple of extra dollars in order to drop a couple of extra pounds, I'm not even talking about shopping at the Farmer's Market or buying all-organic vegetables and produce.

Sure, you can do all that stuff for *extra credit*, but for now let's just get some real food in you for a change and watch how much you light up with all the excess energy and vitality teeming up from within!

If every day you wake up and you love your Tribe, you love yourself and you love your stomach—oh, my, how your life is gonna just keep getting better and better. But don't take my word for it...try it out for yourself!

Progression #11: Love
YOUR NEXT STEP...

DO go easy on your Tribe and give them room to make mistakes as you continue your own personal transformation

Do love yourself and pamper yourself whenever possible

Do love your stomach and treat it to real food on a daily basis

"Your vision will become clear only when you can look into your own heart. Who looks outside, dreams; who looks inside, awakes."
--Carl Jung

PROGRESSION #12:
Create

Create A New Body

What's the point of this entire journey if we're not going to take advantage of this opportunity to create an entirely new life for ourselves, inside and out?!

You now have a far superior understanding of how your body truly works—how it stores and maintains fat, and how it lets go of fat—than the vast majority of humanity will ever have in their whole lives.

As you adopt each of one these progressions into your lifestyle, your body will begin reflecting a completely different reality...a reality where fat-burning Glucagon is the Big Man on Campus and his sidekick, the appetite-suppressing, energy-stimulating hormone Leptin, is his Right-Hand Man!

Letting go of your sugar and Mega-Sugar habit isn't just the best possible way to make a triumphant return to your Ideal Body...it's the *only* way!

The progressions of the *Low Carb Revolution* will take you to your initial destination, but why stop there?

We have a saying in Spanish, "Que las montanas desean, los valles no vean." This translates to: "What the mountains desire, the valleys can't even see."

As you continue into Part Two of this book and you become more and more connected with your incredible body, you may start to discover places you want to take it that you never imagined possible.

Of course it's a noble and valuable journey to return

294

to our Ideal Body. But why stop working on ourselves there?! Why not really create the body we truly desire?!

"To practice any art, no matter how well or badly, is a way to make your soul grow. So do it."
—Kurt Vonnegut

Express Yourself

If you desire the lean, muscular look that I have developed, then start dancing...and keep dancing! I deliberately cultivated a dancer's body, adn so can you! To start with, stay away from the gym, don't lift any weights and don't ever go for a pointless "run"! (I strongly believe the only reasons two reasons to run are because something dangerous is chasing us or we're trying to catch something—like a plane or a train or our true love!)

Instead of "working out", go play! Take up social dancing. Learn the two-step, salsa, rumba, cha cha, lambada, bachata, tango...the more, the better. You'll meet people and you'll have fun and you'll naturally slim down your body by expressing it through dance.

Or, what the hell, disregard everything I've just said and *do* go lift weights if you're pulled in that direction.

The woman in the picture below is Ernestine Shepherd. She's a 75 year-old grandmother who took up bodybuilding at the ripe old age of 71!

Ernestine does the *opposite* of everything I've just told you! She trains with weights four times a week. She competes in 5K and 10K races, and even runs marathons of over 26 miles while nobody is chasing her! And that path works perfectly for her. Just look at her. She's happy, healthy, eats well and doesn't take any medications whatsoever.

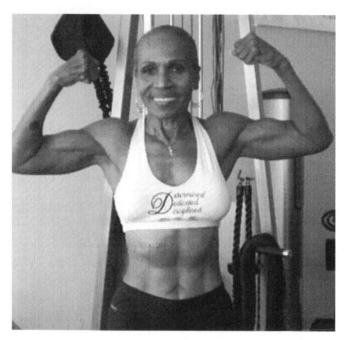

Find your inner Ernestine and let her out to play—whether on the dance floor or (heaven help us, lulz!) at the gym or somewhere in between!

Create A New You

Creating an all new body is one thing—and a good thing, at that. But, again, why stop there?!

What other areas of our life deserve a little more creativity and direction?! Or even a lot more creativity and direction!

As our new, improved, lemon-scented relationship with our body continues to heat up (oh la la!), we'll find ourselves in a position to do more and be more than we've ever been before, to let our light shine so brightly in the world that it's almost blinding. And that's what it's all about, baby!

To get there, we're going to need to color outside the lines. We're going to want to try out new habits and new ways of expressing ourselves. Will that be a little scary at first?! You betcha, but we're gonna do it anyway. Because that's where our growth, our progress, our transformation can be found.

"As you move toward a dream,
the dream moves toward you."
—Julia Cameron

Create More "Art"

As you develop the habit of bringing more creativity into your body and your life, perhaps you might also start bringing more creativity to your *creativity*...discovering new ways to express yourself and let your Inner Artist out to play. When is the last time you wrote a poem...or a short story...or a personal blog post?!

You know that oversized pad of drawing paper tucked away in the gararge?! Why not haul it out and use it for its intended purpose by drawing pictures on it or something?!

Creating art—whether pottery or popsicle sticks or using chainsaws to carve sculptures out of logs—is both a way to connect with the deepest parts of ourselves and a way to reflect the beauty of the creative force in the universe.

As the ebullient cheerleader for creativity, Julia Cameron puts it, "Creativity is God's gift to us. Using our creativity is our gift back to God."

Remember how the point of chopping vegetables is to chop the vegetables and nothing else? So, too, with making art.

The point of creativity is "simply" to be creative. Selling Art, launching a career as an Artist—that's not what we're talking about here at all. It's the *making* of the art, the expressing of ourselves, that matters.

297

And art can be anything at all. Gardening is art. Cooking is art. Collecting bobble-head dolls or first-edition books or coffee mugs that say, "World's Greatest Grandpa" on the side is art. Building your own house is art, as is decorating it, painting it and creatively raising a family in it. Tattoos—both the giving and the receiving of them—are art. Making sweet love down by the river is most definitely art…or, at least it could be and should be!

All of these are merely excuses to create something where there was nothing before. Creating is one of the most profoundly healing activities we can engage in. Creating re-connects your Mind with your Body. Creating brings more beauty into our lives…and into the world. And what could be better than that?!

Progression #12: Create
YOUR NEXT STEP...

DO give yourself permission to express yourself more creatively than ever before in every aspect of your life

DON'T judge or criticize your own art—whatever that art is. Your job as an "artist" (and we are ALL artists!) is to *make* the art, not judge the art!

> *"Art is not about thinking something up. It is the opposite—it's getting something down."*
> —Julia Cameron

PROGRESSION #13:
Wake Up!

The Blue Pill or the Red Pill?

We each have a choice to make in our lives. We must ultimately decide upon one of two paths to take on our journey forward…

One: We can stay asleep. That's the easy choice. And that's certainly the popular choice.

Two: We can wake up. This choice is tougher. Because waking up means taking responsibility for who we are and what we are doing with ourselves and our life.

If we make the second choice, if we take the metaphorical Red Pill that will awaken us from the "Matrix", then our life will be forever changed.

Our life will become an *ongoing process* of waking up. Waking up to our potential, waking up to our mission here and, ultimately, waking up our Ideal Self and letting her out to play in the world! Make no mistake, *the way we take the Red Pill and wake ourselves up is by letting go of excess sugars and excess carbs.* For these are the culprits that have kept us asleep and numb and unaware all these years.

Every time we reach for a roll, a breadstick or a bowl of oatmeal, we move back in the direction of falling asleep once again.

Do rolls, breadsticks and bowls of oatmeal taste good? Fo sho! But that's not the point. The point is whether we prefer the temporary bliss of the sugar-induced Insulin rush that pushes us back towards our heavy slumbers...or whether we desire the energy, vitality and productivity of continuing to wake up and letting our light shine in the world.

> *"People who habitually consume wheat products become crabby, foggy and tired after just a couple of hours of not having a wheat product, often desperately searching for any crumb or morsel to relive the pain ."*
> —William Davis, MD

The Outer Journey

I so admire you for reaching this stage of our journey together.

You've weathered a fair bit of science and nutrition and even some simple mathematics (egads!) in order to reach this stage. Along the way you've been given the keys behind how our body stores and maintains fat, as well as a series of manageable progressions that will help you let go of your excess weight and belly fat, making a much-deserved return to your natural state and your birthright of your Ideal Body.

The *Low Carb Revolution* is not a diet, it's a lifestyle. It's a sustainable eating plan that will carry you into a scenic and productive future.

Remember that you always have a powerful ally and supporter on your team in the form of the accompanying Audio Affirmations. The more often you play the positive messages of the double-tracked mp3 that I gave you while you go about other aspects of your life, the more its guidance and wisdom will sink into each and every cell of your body.

And remember that I am always on your side and I am just a mouse-click away. Contact me anytime with your comments, questions, success stories or tales about your vacation in Corfu at my personal email addfress: **zombiejohn@gmail.com**.

Everything we've accomplished together until now has been deliberately designed to help our bodies wake up and get here through the foods we consume and the way we move our bodies through the physical space around us.

Now it's time to change gears and turn our investigations inward as we continue our progress towards our ultimate destination.

The Inner Journey

In Part Two we're going inside ourselves...and we're going *deep*. Although from now on we'll be concerning ourselves primarily with the inner workings of our brains, our future success in changing our personal habits still depends upon the energy and vitality available to our bodies...so I recommend not straying far from the principles and best practices we've already learned.

Dip back into Part One now and again to remind yourself that even though you know what to do, you still need to do it!

As Stephen Covey says, "To know, and not to do, is not to know." (It's kinda think-y, but once it sinks in, it's profound!)

Our goal always remains the same...to clear the blocks and obstacles in our Body (Part One) and the negative thoughts and habits in our Mind (Part Two) in order to get out of our own way and allow our Inner Self to finally emerge into the light of day.

I refer to this process as Waking Up, but other cultures have other names for it. In the Hawaiian healing tradition of Huna, they describe this process as, "Remembering who we are".

In Hawaii the shaman (or healer) is known as the Kahuna. And the Kahuna believes that we are all born with a connection to the universal life force, to the Gods and the spirits of the natural world. But then, at about the age of 6 or 7 or 8, because of school or life or for whatever reason, we all fall asleep. Most of us stay asleep for the rest of our lives.

The Kahuna, meanwhile, manages to wake up and "remember who he is"...and then he goes around to the other members of his Tribe and helps them wake up when they're ready.

It took me years of effort and exploration and journeying, but I finally woke up.

And now I've come back for you! If you've made it this far in the *Low Carb Revolution*, then I believe are most definitely ready to wake up...and, indeed, are well on your way to doing so!

Let's keep going. Let's bring it home together in the pages ahead. Let's bring your brilliant, powerful, beautiful, unstoppable Inner Self to play!

Progression #13: Wake Up
YOUR NEXT STEP...

DO make it your intention to wake up and allow your highest, Inner Self to emerge from deep within you so you can finally achieve the success you desire and deserve

DO ask yourself if eating a particular food will give you a temporary, sugar-induced Insulin bliss and then start to put you back to sleep...or if it will serve to help wake you up!

DO play the Audio Affirmations I created to help you succeed in the background as often as possible!

DO consider helping yourself Wake Up further still by writing a book of your own describing how you've overcome the challenges and obstacles in your life.

The Low Carb Revolution by John McLean

*"The best way to make your dreams come true is
to wake up."*
—Paul Valery

The Low Carb Revolution by John McLean

The 13 Progressions of the Low Carb Revolution

1) Eat as much as you want

2) Avoid Excess Sugars

3) Avoid Wheat Products

4) Drink Alcohol in Moderation

5) Avoid Processed Carbs

6) Avoid Drinking Sugars & Carbs

7) Avoid Natural Carbs

8) Mind your pH

9) Mix It Up

10) Cook It Yourself

11) Love

12) Create

13) Wake Up

"If you're not failing every now and again, it's a sign you're not doing anything very innovative."
—Woody Allen

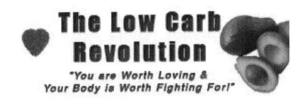

The Low Carb Revolution

*"You are Worth Loving &
Your Body is Worth Fighting For!"*

Part Two:
"Losing Weight is
a Love Story!"

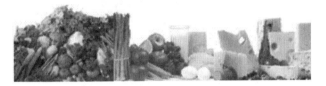

*"Life is either a daring
adventure, or nothing!"*
—Helen Keller

SECRET #1:
"Water Doesn't Boil at 211 Degrees"

The Adventure of a Lifetime!

Welcome to Part Two of the *Low Carb Revolution*! It's my privilege to continue guiding you step-by-step down a path leading to your goal of losing excess pounds easily, naturally and permanently so you can return to your ideal body weight.

Along the way, we'll revisit some of the core beliefs you may have picked up over the years about being overweight—stories you've been telling yourself over and over again about how "difficult" it is to lose weight or how you just can't find the time or energy to shake your booty.

We'll go behind the scenes into our Mind and Body, discovering how a surprising amount of our daily behaviors and activities are merely *habits*. We'll also learn that the primary way we can make lasting changes in our life...weight, smoking, financial success, etc....is by *changing* our habits.

And I'll persist in challenging you all along the way to repair and heal your relationship with your beautiful body!

You'll eventually come to understand how your mind and your body have probably been working *against* each other for a long time now to create the excess weight you've been forced to carry around. And ultimately you'll be among a select group of people who've learned how to get mind *and* body working together again to create harmony and wholeness and bliss in every aspect of your life going forward.

"Winning is a habit.
Unfortunately, so is losing."
—Vince Lombardi

State Change

What we're ultimately after here is helping you create your own personal State Change—one of the most powerful forces in human society as well as in nature.

People have long been fascinated by the very concept of a state change...you know, the transformation of one thing into another.

Caterpillars most famously do this, undergoing a complete state change into a butterfly. Similarly, Dr. Jekyl turned into Mr. Hyde. And in books and movies, humans commonly undergo state changes into Vampires...or Zombies...or Mutants...or even Wizards!

Of course, we humans didn't invent the concept of state changes. As always, the natural world led the way.

Take, for example, the most abundant substance on our planet: water. When water freezes and changes its state from liquid to ice it can sink the largest ships afloat. Yet when water boils and changes its state to steam...entire civilizations and empires arise!

The Industrial Revolution was built on the shoulders of steam, the state that water changes into when you heat it to the boiling point.

Everything in that era was powered by steam— railroads, factory motors, engines of construction and ships. They'd still be digging the Panama Canal today if it weren't for steam.

Even in our current high-tech, computerized,

modern day a-go-go world, simply heating up water until it boils and makes a state change into steam, which then turns a turbine to generate electricity or force, remains the most widespread and important source of power available to mankind.

You would probably imagine that nuclear-powered vessels are among the most complicated systems ever built? If so, you'd be rightl.

Yet, at the same time, the twin nuclear reactors of the most advanced submarine or aircraft carrier in the world fundamentally do only one thing—*heat up water and turn it into steam!* It's the steam created by the heat of the nuclear reactors that drives the propellers and generates the electricity that powers every other system on the entire vessel.

Now stay with me here, because this has *everything* to do with losing weight!

Why A Watched Pot Never Boils

Alright, so how do you turn water into steam? It's pretty straightforward, really. You just heat up the water to 212 degrees Fahrenheit (or 100 degrees Celsius, whichever comes first!) and, voila, the water boils.

Okay, okay….it's not actually quite that simple!

It turns out there's *not* a direct temperature progression once you start heating up water. You don't simply apply heat and observe the temperature of the water rise from, say, 209 degrees to 210 and then 211 and then, finally, the magical boiling point of 212 degrees. Nope, that's just not the way it works. Here's what truly happens…

You start heating the aforementioned water. Eventually it gets to 209 and then 210 and then 211. So it's at 211 and you add more heat…

And it's still at 211…211…211…

So you add even *more* heat, and it's still at 211...211...211 (and you suddenly realize this is why a watched pot never boils!) and the water stubbornly remains at 211...211...211—and you're still adding heat and adding heat and the energy builds and builds and then finally...

It hits 212—and the water's BOILING! And that's what a State Change is!

Nature has set it up so that a seemingly disproportionate amount of energy goes into that last tiny, little degree!

Even when the water is already at 211 degrees and seems sooooo close to success, a lot, *a lot*, a **LOT** of energy still has to be added before it makes the State Change to 212 degrees and begins to boil.

Naturally, the exact same paradigm applies to us.

The Final Degree

All great achievement in our lives—and, believe me, returning to your Ideal Body will be one of the great achievements of your life—involve going through a similar state change.

Every New Year's Eve, gazillions of Americans fashion brand new resolutions for themselves. Resolutions like starting an online business, learning to ride a horse or shedding some lbs.

In the days that follow they pour a little (or even a lot) of energy into their new goal and before long they've got some momentum! Suddenly things are heating up.

They feel soooo close to reaching their goal...209 degrees...210...211!

But then "disaster" strikes: 211...211...211...211... 211...211...

When the "water" doesn't start boiling the very next second, they fear something's gone terribly wrong!

Sometimes they tell themselves a *story* that their plan didn't work or that it's all their fault or they're lazy or don't deserve success — and they just give up.

They were merely one degree away from succeeding and they just quit on themselves!

The entire second half of the *Low Carb Revolution* was designed to heat YOU up to the point where you're ready to make a state change of your own, to the point where you can finally decide to make the beautiful leap from being caught up in a Fat Food Lifestyle and instead learn how to *slow down and live.*

At times during our travels just ahead you may actually feel your internal "temperature" rise degree by degree. At other times you may feel that "nothing" at all is happening deep within you — as if you've reached 211 degrees and now you're "stuck" there!

But you're not stuck...you're exactly where you need to be!

Let me say that again, because it's one of the most profoundly important concepts underlying the work we still have left before us...

Wherever you are now is exactly where you need to be!

If you've finished the 13 Keys and the 13 Progressions, then you already know *exactly* what to do in order to lose the weight you desire.

Now it's just a question of getting yourself to do it. That's why from now on we're gonna just keep applying the heat! Hopefully we're on the same page — so now let's go deeper!

"What we call failure is not the falling down, but the staying down"
— Mary Pickford

It's Story Time!

Once upon a time...there was a guy who smoked more cigarettes than anybody else in the whole wide world. Because at any given moment in time there has to be *somebody* who smokes the most, right?!

Just like there has to be somebody in the world who's the tallest and somebody who's the oldest and the best at water-skiing and the world's #1 grandfather and whatnot.

If you've ever been around cigarette smokers, then you know that the hard-core ones can go through as much as two full packs a day! (I know, disgusting, right?!) Well, ha-ha! Because this guy played in a whole different league. He smoked their entire daily allotment of two packs before lunch. Every single day.

By the end of each day he'd finished off up to FIVE PACKS of cigarettes! Nope, that's not a typo! 5 entire packs. A day. This guy—and let's just go ahead and call him "ME"!—basically bought and smoked an entire CARTON of cigarettes *every other day!*

I was...drum roll, please!...the Heaviest Smoker on Planet Earth! Yup, good times!

For years and years (and years!) I engineered my entire life—personally, professionally, creatively and romantically—in such a way that I was able to smoke almost *constantly* from the time I dragged myself out of uneasy slumbers like Gregor Samsa every morning until the moment I fell back into bed each night, exhausted, depleted and drained from the smoke and toxins of nearly 100 cigarettes in my system.

For most of those years, I didn't even dare *dream* what it would feel like to achieve Escape Velocity from my daily personal hell of smoking.

Like so many others, I was *sleep-walking* through life but didn't even know I was asleep.

311

I couldn't begin to imagine what possible combination of miracles might take place in order to transform me — the Heaviest Smoker on Planet Earth — into a permanent non-smoker. But somehow it did happen!

Somehow I did ultimately make that leap, that transition, that unlikely transmogrification back to my natural state and birthright as a non-smoker!

But the most amazing part was that all the time and energy I invested into discovering how and why habits are formed and how to make the complicated state change from smoker to non-smoker gave me an unexpected understanding into another important issue in my life: my weight.

At the same time that I was smoking all those cigarettes, I also subsisted largely on a Fat Food diet of Krap, while moving my body so little that eventually I turned into an almost 270 lb. blob.

But within a year of finally letting go of cigarettes, I used the very same hard-won knowledge about how we are run by our habits and how our habits are run by our body to transform myself — yet another beautiful state change! — from being Jabba the Hutt's understudy to what turned out to be my ideal body weight of 189 pounds.

Which is a nice, lean weight for a fellow who stands 6'3" tall. Using the principles and learnings that I shared with you in Part One of the *Low Carb Revolution*, I easily and naturally lost 80 pounds — almost *one-third* of my entire body weight.

Now 189 lbs. also just happens to be the exact same amount I weighed as a 17 year-old senior in high school...and yet I am (at least according to my own teenaged children) approximately 2000 years old right now.

But I'm getting ahead of myself! Let's go back to our

story...

My "Little" Smoking Problem

Unearthing the Rosetta Stone to resolve my "little" smoking problem started out as mere wishful thinking, then grew into a part-time hobby, and finally occupied me day and night for the better part of two endless years.

Once I had decided that I was going to do whatever it took to figure out why I smoked cigarettes and what I could possibly do to get rid of my nearly 5 pack per day habit, I decided to go ALL the way down the Rabbit Hole.

In order to dedicate myself to research on negative habits and how to change them, I abruptly quit my successful career in outside Advertising Sales—where I deliberately worked out in the field, on my own and without direct supervision so that I could furiously chain-smoke between every sales call!

To keep myself in cigarettes, I took a part-time job as a Strip Club Disc Jockey, since gentlemen's clubs still openly allowed smoking in a town where indoor smoking was otherwise strictly forbidden. (My only prerequisite for the new gig was that I be able to smoke on the job—since I quite literally couldn't go *10 minutes* without a cigarette, much less an entire 10-hour DJ shift!)

Mad Scientist Mode

Outside of chain-smoking my way through a few DJ shifts at local strip clubs (again, you can't make this stuff up!) per week, I became a virtual recluse.

I spent every free moment of my time holed up in my bedroom behind a mountain of books on addiction and biology, listening to audio recordings on motivation and psychology while scribbling reams of detailed notes...amidst overflowing ashtrays and smoke so thick I had to permanently remove the battery from the fire detector thingie over the door to keep it from going off all the time!

I went into what my friends jovially termed "Mad Scientist" mode, cutting out all the extracurricular activities from my life—you know, "useless" stuff like exercise and eating properly and dating!

Two years passed. Two Christmases and two Thanksgivings...two sets of everyone's birthday and two sets of all the other holidays, big and small.

Bit by bit, piece by piece, over hill and over dale, and well past grandmother's house, during those twenty-four months I managed to solve the most complicated problem I had ever personally faced.

Degree by degree, I learned how raise my temperature from within: 209...210...211...211...211...211... 211...211...211... 211...211...211...211...211...

Until...finally, two full-time years into my endeavor, long past the point where many would've abandoned ship, it happened, I reached...212 Degrees!

When at last I emerged into the light of day, I had discovered how to create my own STATE CHANGE!

The water was a-boiling...and I was no longer a-smokin'! I discovered how to go from nearly 5 packs of cigarettes per day to ZERO—literally overnight! And I did it without any useless pills, patches or other outside assistance from Big Pharmacy!

By reframing the way my Mind and my Body processed the entire cigarette smoking experience, I learned how to send a message to every single cell that I no longer wished to smoke cigarettes.

And once my cells got the message, the change was instantaneous and permanent.

I haven't had a cigarette since that magical day some

years ago nor have I ever felt the slightest pang or desire to ever have one again.

Indeed, my past incarnation as the Heaviest Smoker on Planet Earth now seems so dim, distant and inaccessible that it's almost like it was somebody else puffing away on those cigarettes all those years and not me!

> *"You cannot keep determined*
> *people from success"*
> —Mary Kay Ash

A Double Rainbow!

When I had first entered my "Mad Scientist" phase, I wasn't even thinking about my excess weight. Seriously, returning to my Ideal Body was nowhere to be found on my To Do list.

I just sort of accepted the fact that I had somehow become a chubby monkey and let it go at that. But in a way, solving the supremely difficult problem of smoking cessation turned into the perfect proving ground for the radical new theories about mind and body and habit change that I had developed during my years of isolated, focused study and research.

After all, cigarette smoking is a pretty complicated problem. And it's terribly easy to verify your success.

Even on a weight-loss program that really works, like the *Low Carb Revolution*, it still takes some weeks and months to naturally return to your ideal weight. However, with smoking cigarettes, you pretty much know if your theory was correct and you've succeeded at helping yourself or someone else let go of cigarettes within an *hour* — two at the most!

Heaven knows that if my mind-body habit theories weren't correct then I personally wouldn't have been able to go fifteen minutes without smoking, much less, oh, the rest of my life! But it *did* work. I did go from smoking 5 (that's *cinco*, for my Spanish-speaking amigos!) packs of cigarettes one day to absolutely zero the next day without any sickness, pain or cravings.

So what I want to share with you are some all-new theories of how our mind and body can work together (or, sadly, for most of us, work *against* one another) to allow us to do amazing things like dropping excess pounds and returning easily and naturally to our Ideal Body!

"The most terrifying thing in the world is to accept oneself completely"
— Carl Jung

Thanks for Playing!

Once again, thank you for joining me on this leg of the wonderful journey we're taking together! I'm well-aware you have all sorts of other obligations and distractions around you — work, family, life, checking your Facebook status every 10 minutes, lulz! — as well as people, technology, advertising, entertainment and even pets constantly competing for your attention.

I feel privileged to be your guide as you continue moving towards a return to your birthright and natural state of health, energy and well-being.

The United States is now the fattest country on the entire planet — with nearly 7 out of every 10 adults overweight or obese.

By the Center for Disease Control's most conservative estimates, approximately 1 out of every 3 Americans now alive will become a full-fledged diabetic within the next generation.

Oh by the way, developing diabetes will substantially lower their quality of life and, on average, chop almost a decade off their lifespan.

A growing number of families now spend more on pills and medications to fix their Fat Food lifestyle problems than they spend on food itself!

In just the past decade, the amount of money we've handed over to Big Pharmacy in the United States has more than *doubled*—rising from just over $100 billion per year in 2000 to a staggering $250 billion in 2010!

Just to put this in perspective for you, Americans spend $500 billion each year in total for all our food expenditures!

This means our pill budget alone currently adds up to fully HALF of our entire food budget...and our pill expenditures just continue to rise and rise, while each year we spend a little bit less on food itself.

Clearly, the drive thru, Fat Food lifestyle doesn't work...unless, of course, you're a stockholder in one of the multi-national corporations behind Big Diet. Even in the economic downturn of the past few years, the stocks of fast food chains and Big Diet are rising faster as our collective blood pressure.

Meanwhile, spending half of our annual food budget on pills is itself hardly normal.

Our natural state is Health, not sickness! Hippocrates, the father of medicine, advised us: "Nutrition shall be your medicine."

A "normal" percentage of our annualfood budget to donate to the coffers of Big Pharmacy is approximately 0%! Instead of death by Fat Food, maybe it's time we learn how to...

Slow Down...and Live!

And by "live", I mean both to live longer, to have more years of fun on this incredibly diverse planet, and to live it up and enjoy our time here more than ever before!

The Low Carb Revolution by John McLean

*"Every time I see an adult on a
bicycle, I no longer despair for
the future of the human race."*
—H.G. Wells

SECRET #2:
"We Don't Run Our Habits...Our Habits Run US!"

Another Day at the Office

One day my friend Lisa was driving to the grocery store when her cell phone rang. An old school chum she hadn't spoken to in like *forever* was on the line. As she chatted with her friend, Lisa kept driving, more focused on her phone conversation than on her destination.

After a good 45 minutes of talking and driving, Lisa realized she had arrived at her goal. Lisa finished up the call as she pulled into the vast parking lot of the office building where she worked.

Curiously, there's wasn't a single other car parked outside her office building.

Even more curiously, Lisa looked down at herself and it slowly sank in that instead of being dressed for work, she sported warm-up bottoms and fuzzy slippers.

Finally it dawned on her that it was Saturday! The office was closed. Then she remembered she wasn't heading toward work at all when she'd started out. Rather she'd been on her way to the grocery store when the call from her old schoolmate distracted her attention away from where she was going.

With a weary sigh, Lisa turned the car around and began the long drive home.

Now here's an interesting question for you…

While Lisa's Mind was busy enjoying the telephone conversation with her friend, WHO exactly was driving her car?

Was That My Exit?

Maybe you've had a similar experience. You're driving, say, from one end of town to another, and as you drive you get lost in your thoughts. Like we all do.

Perhaps you're thinking about how Jenkins over in Accounting is really getting on your nerves these days...and that leads you to pondering whether it's finally time to leave the firm and find a new job...which causes you to wonder whether you should finally get out of the widget business altogether and change career paths...which leads you to dream of leaving the rat race behind entirely and moving to an obscure Hawaiian island to build custom surf boards for left-handed surfers—and suddenly you notice a sign saying "EXIT 245A" zooming past the car window and you're jolted back into the NOW!

"OhmyGod, was that my exit?!" you exclaim! With a start, you realize that "you" have been piloting some 4000-odd lbs. of metal, glass and rubber at over 60 mph down the freeway without being consciously "aware" of what you were doing!

Instead, you were completely lost in your thoughts—imagining yourself at your current job (blech!), imagining yourself in Hawaii (yay!), imagining selling your first custom surfboard (ka-ching!)—and you have absolutely no recollection of how you go to Exit 245A so quickly!

In fact, as you think back on the 20-minute drive you just made, you realize that while you do have memories of the *thoughts* you were thinking during the drive, you have no memories at all of the journey itself.

So your brain was caught up in your thoughts and daydreams and it clearly wasn't driving your car. And yet you still arrived at your destination safely.

But *somebody* had to be driving your car! If it wasn't you, again, then who the hell was it?!

Who's Driving The Car?

Once we do it enough, driving becomes a habit. Habits are actions we've learned to do so well that we no longer need to think about the steps that go into them. In other words, habits are activities we can do on auto-pilot.

If you remember back when you first learned to drive a car, it seemed as if were so many different details to watch out for and pay attention to. It took 100% of your focus and attention just to parallel park. At times you probably feared you'd never master all the complicated aspects of driving a car.

And yet, over time, you probably got so good at driving that you can now get in the car, turn it on, think of your destination—work, grocery store, grandma's house—and then pretty much forget about it after that.

Nowadays, we can (and usually do) spend our entire drivetime talking on the phone, thinking about our life, listening to music/audio books or carrying on a lively conversation with someone else in the car—each of which are activities performed by our mind.

Since we know how to drive a car by *habit*, that means we no longer need our mind to focus on the action steps for shifting gears or making a left hand turn or flipping somebody off when they cut in front of us.

This means our mind has pretty much *nothing* to do during drives except for thinking about stuff, talking, listening to music, etc.

A habit is anything we do without needing to think

about how to do it.

Smokers don't have to remember to smoke. When I smoked nearly 5 packs per day all those years, it never once happened that I reached the end of the day and realized with a shock that I had completely forgotten to smoke a single cigarette for the entire day!

No, I was in the HABIT of smoking. My smoking habit ran itself, without any additional input on my part. Every few minutes I would just light up another cigarette and smoke the entire thing without any conscious awareness of doing so.

And you do the same with all the many habits in your life.

You are (hopefully!) in the habit of brushing your teeth regularly. Now once you decide to brush your teeth, you don't have to pause and figure out each step. You don't pick up the toothbrush and stare it while wondering which end to brush your teeth with. You don't need to waste precious synapses figuring out how to open the toothpaste tube and get the stuff onto the end of the toothbrush. You don't have to figure out how to apply the paste to your teeth and so.

You learned all of these steps as a kid, and you learned them so well that for the rest of your life you don't ever need to think about how to brush your teeth again. Brushing your teeth has become a habit for you.

In fact, most people make even the decision of *when* to brush their teeth a habit so they don't even have to think about the best times to run the habit of brushing their teeth! They brush their teeth at regular times like first thing in the morning, right before bed, fresh out of the shower and so on.

They "automate" the times they brush their teeth or run many other habits in exactly the same way I'm encouraging you to "automate" eating a healthy, low-carb breakfast and lunch each day to help the pounds continue to drop off.

Now if you land a new job, the first time or three you drive to work you may have to consult a map or ask directions to figure out where the hell you're going. But after just a few repetitions your amazing brain will learn how to reach this new destination so well that you literally won't have to ever think about it with your "mind" anymore.

All you'll need to do is "tell yourself" in some form or another at the start of your journey where you're going and then your mind is free to do whatever it likes until you get there. At that point, driving to work or other destinations becomes automatic.

Of course, at other times we inadvertently *omit* this little step of telling ourselves where to go!

That's how Lisa made the long drive to her office on a Saturday and how we might end up taking the freeway exit that leads to our house when we meant to continue two more exits up the road and stop by the grocery store to pick up a gallon of milk on the way home.

How We Learn Habits

When we first learn any new activity, we absolutely do need our mind to get the ball rolling. If you have no musical experience and you decide to take up the banjo, you don't just sit down and start playing that creepy tune from "Deliverance" from the get-go.

No, your mind needs weeks and months of learning where the notes are and how to play them, and it needs years and more of focus and practice in order to learn a variety of songs and tunes.

Yet if you keep going down this road, eventually you have to think less and less as you play the banjo and you can simply just "play" without needing to remember what notes to play next.

To get really good at a musical instrument—to get to the point where you no longer need to think about what and how to play—you're going to need to spend a lot of time practicing.

Canadian journalist and bon vivant (why not?!) Malcolm Gladwell postulates that becoming a true master of any activity—whether banjo or golf or flying jet fighters off an aircraft carrier—requires some 10,000 hours of practice.

I'll do the math for you: that's about 5 entire years of full-time, 40 hours per week, focused practice.

Or, more commonly, 10 years of moderately serious, 3 hours per day, 7 days a week practice.

Of course, that's what is required to become a world-class zen-master *virtuoso* at something. We can and do turn some of our simpler behaviors into habits in as little as a single repetition.

You only have to stick a fork in an electrical socket once in your life...and you'll remember not to do that again from now on!

Whether it takes just a single trial or 10,000 hours to master a given activity, *eventually* it will become a habit for us and we'll no longer to need to stop and think about how to do it.

To return to our earlier questions…

Who was driving Lisa's car as she drove 45 minutes in the wrong direction while absorbed in a telephone conversation? Who is driving your car when you reach a destination on the other side of town without any particular memories of how you got there?

If our minds aren't in charge of our habits, who is?

Meanwhile Back in the Laboratory

Recall that I had previously spent two long, focused years in Mad Scientist mode, hidden away in my "laboratory" researching and studying the subject of habit, especially.

Following that I spent an additional three dedicated years learning how to organize and share with others what I had learned about habits in order to make a difference in their lives—to help them quit smoking, overcome trauma or fall back in love with themselves so they could lose the weight that's been holding them back.

At first I was concerned exclusively with the deep, complicated habit of smoking cigarettes, but I later expanded my horizons to include all the many varieties of behaviors we do entirely out of habit. Because we can get in the habit of doing almost anything…even shitty things that we don't particularly want to do!

We can rather easily get in the habit eating Krap from McTacoHut Drive-Thru on our way to work each morning. We no longer have to think about what to do for breakfast, we just go there.

This is why I encourage you to purposefully "automate" one or more meals each day—which means to create a habit of consuming foods that serve your goal of reducing belly fat rather than contribute to it.

We can get in the habit of sitting down to watch a little (on average, a "little" translates to more than 6 hours per evening in America!) TV after work. Sure, each night of the week the shows themselves are different, but the habit of watching hours of television every day rarely varies. We can get in the habit of cracking our knuckles, twisting our hair, picking at our skin, waking up to eat a midnight snack and a thousand other activities—some of them good for us and others not so much.

For several years I closely studied all the existing theories of how we form habits and how to change them.

Many of these theories about habits were quite

wordy and clever, and they were often created by people with a dizzying pile of advanced degrees and certifications.

But none of these theoretical approaches to habit change were of the slightest help back when I was trying to achieve Escape Velocity from my not-at-all-theoretical habit of smoking half a carton of cigarettes every day.

I should add that even before my two year-long descent into the study of habits, I already had a strong foundation in the science of how our brains work—both the classical and alternative models.

I was already a formally trained hypnotist, having been trained and certified by the late, great American hypnotist, Gil Boyne.

And I was a Master Practitioner (a somewhat lofty level, as these things go) in the related discipline of Neuro-Linguistic Programming, having studied with one of the foremost writers and teachers of NLP in the world, Robert Dilts, along with his colleague Judith Delozier...the same duo who a few years earlier had taught motivational rockstar Tony Robbins the exact same material at the exact same location at the University of California at Santa Cruz.

Both hypnosis and NLP have their own theories and techniques for changing habits—which sometimes work and sometimes don't.

But I really couldn't waste my time with "sometimes". If I was ever going to successfully change my own deeply entrenched habit of smoking, it was all or nothing...it had to work completely and totally!

Finally, after a great deal of searching and experimentation, I made the discovery that changed everything. I made a discovery that nothing else had prepared me for.

And the discovery was that, contrary to what almost

every expert and every discipline was telling me, our habits are NOT run by our minds at all!

Just think about it observationally...

If our habits were run by our minds, then we could change them just by changing our thinking—which, of course, is exactly the advice that the lion's share of "experts" out there are selling us, sorry, I meant to say "telling" us, haha! It turns out our habits are run by another part of us.

A part of us we regularly tend to be cut off and disconnected from—which is why it took me so long to realize what was going on.

Let's cut to the chase, shall we?!

Our Habits Are Run By Our Body

Our old friend-slash-nemesis, our beautiful *body*, is back again!

And the truth of is—despite decades of the motivational "wisdom" about thinking our way to success—*our habits are not run by our mind at all, but entirely and exclusively by our body.*

When people learn things really well—whether it's a musical instrument or dance or sports—their conscious mind cannot possibly track and predict all the possible variables that going into this complicated behavior.

But their *body* can and does.

When Michael Jordan played basketball, he didn't stop and think about where to step and which foot to jump off and how to hold the ball. He just let his body take over and it figured out how to defy gravity and seemingly fly through the air on the way to a spectacular dunk.

Although a habit like driving to work is not quite as attention-grabbing as watching Baryshnikov dance, both are examples of the same thing: actions that have been learned so well that they are carried out by the body without calling on the mind.

Indeed, if you want to ruin any artist's performance, just get them to start *thinking* about it with their mind rather than merely doing it with their body and the whole thing will immediately fall apart!

Of course, the mind has some small input. It can help us decide whether or not we're going to run one of our habits. For example, when we're about to drive somewhere, it's the responsibility of the mind to tell our body where to go.

If we forget to communicate this important piece of information to our body, it's forced to guess.

Since our body isn't really even aware of what's going on in the outside world (much more on this just ahead), as often as not the mind guesses wrong—which is how my friend Lisa ended up driving all the way to her office building on a Saturday rather than to the local grocery store or wherever it was she was going that morning.

For sure your mind can temporarily override the habits carried out by your body—the key word being *temporarily*. Most smokers can easily quit smoking just by thinking about it...for one day!

Some time back my friend Marcia resolved to end her habit of drinking Dr. Pepper from morning til night. She got herself all "psyched up" to stop drinking Dr. Pepper and then consciously, deliberately and purposefully kept herself from drinking a single one for 17 straight days.

By that time, she reckoned she had kicked her habit through force of mind and willpower.

Then one day she was driving somewhere and looked down to see that she was sipping from a large fountain drink of Dr. Pepper! She glanced in the rear view mirror and saw the receding outline of a fast food joint in the distance.

Apparently, while lost in thought (a common theme when we get into cars, huh?!) her *body* drove her through the nearest Fat Food drive thru and bought itself a Dr. Pepper, which her body was now happily enjoying!

By the time Marcia's mind even noticed what she was doing, the Dr. Pepper was already half finished. And you already know this story ends. Before long, Marcia was back to chugging Dr. Peppers not just at the prescribed hours of 10, 2 and 4 but also at every possible moment in between!

Each New Year's day, millions of Americans resolve to finally get in shape. And so what do they do? They "will" themselves with their minds to get up early and go for a run. And maybe they actually *do* go out for a run. But running is not a habit for them. Yet. It's just something they decided to do one morning.

Running only becomes a habit when they no longer have to think about it—when their body gets up seemingly on its own and heads out the door for a run and their mind only notices they were running when the run is winding down and it's time to think about what activity to do next.

Is this making sense for you?! I know this is probably *nothing* like any theory of understanding habits you've ever been exposed to before...but if you continue down this road with me and really understand how the mind and the BODY work together, I assure you that changing your eating habits (or any of your habits, for that matter) will become so much easier than you've ever believed possible!

When you first encountered the 13 Progressions, implementing all of them in your daily life might have seemed a bit daunting, even overwhelming.

I guarantee you that by the time you finish Part Two of the *Low Carb Revolution*, you're gonna be saying,

"Oh, yessir, I can do that, easy peasy!"

> *"Knowledge is only a rumor until you get it*
> *in your muscles"*
> —Robert Dilts

"Just Do It!"

Now habits aren't restricted to negative behaviors like chewing tobacco, stopping at the pub on the home from work every day or regularly eating processed Krap instead of actual food.

Really *any* activity we do that we no longer need to think about while we're doing it can be classified as a habit. Any task we can "automate" becomes a habit.

My friend Ames is an incredible hairstylist. Back when she was in beauty school, her mind deliberately guided, analyzed and judged every single snip of her shears...that was how she learned to cut hair. In those days before I decided to start shaving my head, I had long, luxurious locks of golden curls flowing to my shoulders. (Well, at least that's how *I* remember it, lulz!)

In any case, back when Ames was a fledgling hairstylist it took her 45 minutes or longer to cut my hair.

By the time she'd put in her 10,000 hours of absorbing the habit of cutting hair into her body she could do that same haircut in 7 minutes or less. These days Ames can snip away with the speed and artistry of Edward Scissorhands while her mind is actively engaged in conversing with her clients on any and every topic under the sun.

She no longer has to think about cutting hair, it's a habit her body performs effortlessly...leaving her mind free to gossip, which is a good thing indeed because it turns out that gossip is what hairstylists really get paid for and the haircutting and coloring part is just an excuse to get together.

This is key behind Nike's spectacularly successful marketing slogan, "Just DO it!" What Nike is selling is that there is no value in *thinking* about jogging. The point of jogging is to get out and DO it, with your body!

Is *Everything* a Habit?

Some sociologists speculate that upwards of 95% of our daily activities are "automated" and can be categorized as habits.

Most of us are in the habit of waking up at a certain time every weekday morning and getting ready to head to the office or some variation of that theme. After showering and stuff our body drives us to work on auto-pilot. It doesn't even matter if we're still half-asleep or if we're totally distracted by thoughts about the argument we had with our partner the night before since our body knows how to drive our car and knows exactly where we work.

Then we spend a good deal of the day carrying out pretty much the same work-related habits we did yesterday...which are pretty much the same work-related habits we'll do again tomorrow.

Next we return home and, still on auto-pilot, many of us are in the habit of watching television for the proverbial 6 or more hours. Again, the shows vary from day to day, but the habit of watching something on television (or the Internet, no difference) remains the same.

Here's where we're going with all this...the *reason* so many of us live a Fat Food lifestyle isn't because we chose to.

Most of us never decided one way or the other. Eating Krap all the time just became a *habit* while we were busy thinking about other shit! In the past we visited the neighborhood McTacoHut one too many times and our body eventually "learned" this was the place to go when it felt hunger pangs.

Even the executives at the Fat Food franchises know this. By conducting repeated surveys they've learned that more than 80% of all visits to their restaurants are made on "impulse".

That means 8 out of every 10 customers of theirs left home that day without the deliberate intention to head to McTacoHut...their bodies just somehow brought them there without any specific input from their mind about it!

The Trouble With Habits

No doubt, habits are an excellent survival strategy. By learning new tasks so well that our bodies can carry them out for us, that frees up our mind to learn other useful things.

But your body doesn't possess the ability to make a judgment about whether any particular habit it performs is good or bad. That's what your mind is for, making judgments and deciding things.

And this is precisely why our body stubbornly persists in carrying out "negative" behaviors like smoking cigarettes or eating Fat Food that our mind knows for a fact will actually KILL us!

Once more, our body doesn't think about the negative consequences of any our habits because that's the mind's job.

I used to be in the habit of eating Krap every night right before I went to bed. (If you had asked me about it, I would have denied it was a "habit"; instead I convinced myself that I just happened to be hungry every single night before going to bed.)

And since I was in the habit of eating Krap every

night, I never had to decide whether or not to do it. I just wobbled into the kitchen at the appointed hour, parked myself in front of a huge plate of food-shaped chemicals and went to town!

Mind versus Body

Now the biggest challenge in letting go of a negative habit or adopting a positive one is communicating *what we desire to ourselves.*

(Discovering that one "little" part of the equation alone took me years and years...and I continue to explore the implications of this discovery in my life and the lives of the people I work with.)

Communication with ourselves is difficult because our minds are so regularly disconnected from our bodies that there's often virtually no contact between them.

For many of us, our mind and our body aren't even on speaking terms!

The only way I could end up 80 lbs. overweight and smoking an implausible 5 packs of cigarettes per day was by ignoring my body completely. I quite deliberately thought my mind was "all-important" and my body was "stupid" and was just "getting in my way"!

Only as I went through my own personal Couples Counseling did my mind finally learn how to speak body...and my body even learned a few halting words of mind-speak.

Only *then* was I able to begin making serious and lasting changes in my habits and lifestyle.

All the interlocking pieces of my discovery about how our habits are run by our body are precisely what I'll be sharing with you throughout the rest of this book.

Coming up next...in Secret #3 you'll finally learn WHY diets don't work and WHY we rarely lose any lasting weight on them!

> *"The Body often tries to bring our
> attention back to the 'scene of the
> crime' to help us heal it"*
> — Christine Northrup

SECRET #3:
"Your Body is Fighting a Totally Different War"

The Battle In the Pacific

During World War II, the battle in the Pacific was particularly fierce...not only at sea and by air, but also on land. Unlike Europe, there was no single gigantic landmass capable of fielding tank battles and entire armies. Instead, there were islands. Dozens of islands, hundreds of islands — any one of which could prove to be a potential foothold for either side.

The Imperial Japanese Army launched an all-out effort to put as many soldiers on as many islands as possible.

On the smaller islands, these Japanese soldiers were usually ordered to stay hidden and carry out whatever acts of sabotage they could get away with to help derail the Allied war effort. And so they did.

Eventually, of course, the war ended, peace was restored and treaties signed.

Little by little, the pockets Japanese soldiers on the various islands were gathered up and shipped home and life gradually returned to normal. Well, for all but one soldier...

The Most Loyal Soldier

In the spring of 1945, Nazi Germany teetered on the brink of collapse, but the Japanese dug in their heels and had every intention of going down fighting. A young Japanese soldier, 2nd Lieutenant Hiroo Onoda, was given a mission of waging guerilla warfare against the locals on Lubang Island, a smallish island belonging to the Philippines.

His commanding officer, a Major Taniguchi, gave him very specific orders: Under no circumstances was Lt. Onoda to surrender and under no circumstances could he commit suicide.

One afternoon, not long after sneaking onto Lubang Island, Lt. Onoda heard the drone of an American military plane approaching.

He and his men raced through thick foliage and hid beneath a crumbling stone bridge as the plane flew past. Moments later came the tell-tale flutter of propaganda leaflets and a paper shower rained to the ground around them.

Picking up one of the pamphlets, Onoda saw it was printed in Japanese and proclaimed the Great War was over.

The pamphlet said all soldiers had been ordered by the Imperial Japanese Army to immediately cease fighting, lay down their weapon and turn themselves into local authorities, where, the pamphlet asserted, they would be treated with all due respect, blah, blah, blah.

Lt. Onoda crushed the leaflet in his hand and threw it aside with contempt. He'd been warned about these. "A hoax!" Onoda spat.

He thought back to his orders from Major Taniguchi, which specifically commanded him not to surrender, so, well, surrendering was out of the question.

As the sound of the American plane was lost in the distance, Lt. Onoda stood up again. "We will continue fighting," he announced. And so they did.

Week after week, the young Japanese officer and the

three commandos accompanying him eluded detection while cutting phone lines, stealing food and generally wreaking enough havoc to be a nuisance to their enemy, yet without incurring so much wrath that the locals would send a large number of soldiers into the jungle looking for them.

Another plane or two dropped more "Yo, the war is over!" propaganda leaflets, which Onoda pointedly ignored.

Sometimes the locals would spot them in the woods and shout at them, "Go home Japanese soldiers, the war is over!"

Upon which Onoda and his men would shoot at them and then seek shelter further in the woods.

About a year into their mission, one of Onoda's men was shot in the leg by a local farmer. It wasn't a serious wound, but it grew infected and there was nothing they could do to save the soldier's life. After a long, painful night he died of the infection. In the morning, they buried him and moved deeper still into the jungle.

Not long thereafter, one of Onoda's two remaining men ran away in the middle of the night and surrendered to the authorities.

Just a few weeks later, Onoda's sole remaining comrade at arms was shot and killed during a skirmish with local police. Lt. Hiroo Onoda was now left to fend for himself.

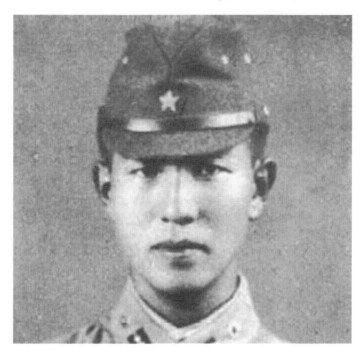

He eventually became something of a legend on the small island. The farmers and authorities knew he was out there somewhere, but sightings were rare and nobody was able to get close enough to the wily soldier to capture him.

From time to time the local authorities would try to lure him out of the jungle, shouting to him that the war was over and he should go home.

Onoda ignored them. Of course. Whenever his resolve weakened, he unfolded his orders from Major Taniguchi and read them again. They were very clear...under no circumstances was he to surrender or take his own life.

And so the loyal Lt. Onoda soldiered on alone in the jungles of tiny Lubang Island.

For twenty-nine years!

The Low Carb Revolution by John McLean

*"Most successful people are ordinary people
with extraordinary determination!"*
—Mary Kay Ash

The End Is Nigh

Let's fast forward nearly three decades...

In early 1974, a globe-trotting Japanese college student set out to find, in no particular order, a giant Panda, the Abominable Snowman and the infamous Lt. Onoda who went off to war and never came back. (Once more, you cannot make this stuff up—this is a 100% true story!)

Against all odds, the young college student tracked down Hiroo Onoda on Lubang Island and spent several days with him in the jungle.

The young student—who hadn't even been born when Lt. Onoda first began his mission—made an effort to persuade the determined soldier the war was over.

Onoda stuck to his guns, insisting that only his commanding officer could order him to surrender. At the same time, Onoda liked the young student and even allowed the kid to take photographs of them together.

Armed with proof that 2nd Lt. Onoda was still alive, the student returned to Japan and appealed directly to the Imperial Japanese Army to find a way to bring home the last remaining soldier from World War II.

Realizing that Onoda wasn't going to be easily persuaded, the Japanese brass took the extraordinary step of tracking down his former commanding officer, Major Taniguchi, who had settled into a quiet life as a bookseller.

Due to his sedentary lifestyle, the Major's old uniform no longer fit him. So the Army commandeered a local tailor and insisted he work around the clock to make a new, more generously sized uniform for the Major.

A Hero's Welcome

In March 1974, Major Taniguchi was airlifted to Lubang Island and after a few days of searching he and his group managed to located the legendary Hiroo Ononda in person.

With the all the formality the former Major could remember from a war career three decades in the past, he officially ordered the younger—although no longer young—man to lay down his arms. Which he summarily did.

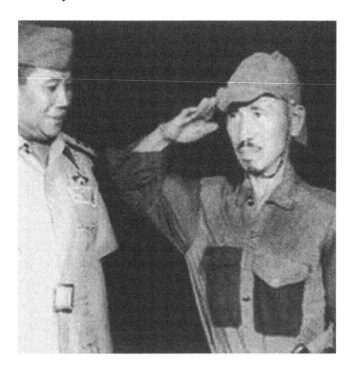

After all these years, the 2nd Lt.'s rifle was still in perfect operating condition. And despite numerous shootouts with locals over the years, he still had 500

rounds of ammunition and several working hand grenades in his possession.

On March 9th, 1974, the war finally ended for Hiroo Onoda, almost THIRTY YEARS after the rest of the world acknowledged it.

His story was front page news around the globe and he returned home to a hero's welcome. Onoda instantly became one of the most popular and beloved figures in Japan.

Songs were written about him, a campaign was launched to encourage him to run for parliment (he graciously declined) and they even made a postage stamp in his honor! The most loyal soldier in history was finally home!

FOOTNOTE: As of mid-2012, former 2nd Lieutenant Hiroo Onoda still remains alive — hale and hearty well into his nineties. I mean, he can't leave this planet because he doesn't have orders to! *Dude is probably gonna outlive us all!*

Our Own Personal War

What does the incredible, true story of this loyal and persistent soldier have to teach us about how to change our negative habits and finally lose our excess belly fat? Well, everything!

Each of our bodies has the dedication and fighting spirit of Lieutenant Hiroo Onoda in it. Once we learn and adopt a habit — whether good, bad or indifferent — our body will ordinarily continue running that habit forever.

The habit stays with us for life until and unless new orders come along.

And not just *any* new orders. Our body has to believe these new orders are "real", otherwise they'll ignore them the way Onoda & Co. ignored the propaganda pamphlets.

If we currently have a negative habit, at a certain

341

point in the past our body got (or *thought* it got...same thing) orders that it was supposed to carry out that habit.

But things change. Life evolves and in our mind we decide we no longer want/need that habit. Yet our body — again, *the part of us that actually carries out the habit* — is utterly unaware of these "new orders" from the mind, so the body keeps soldiering on with the long-time habit.

Our body is actually quite proud of the job its doing of continuing to run this habit against such odds because it still has no idea the war is over!

Let's restate that again, just to make sure it sinks in, because once you grasp this your understanding of how you form and how you can modify your habits will be changed forever.

Our Body continues to run habits that our Mind no longer desires for one reason and one reason only...

Our Body Doesn't Know The War is Over!

Once our body receives its instructions — for example, that it's perfectly okay to eat the fattening, food-shaped chemicals collectively known as Krap — it will keep performing that mission for...ever!

Lt. Onoda followed the orders he was given and didn't have any *opinion* about whether his orders were good or sound or reasonable.

They were his orders, like them or not, and he intended to carry them out, period.

Our body does the same thing. It doesn't have the wherewithal to judge or decide if, say, smoking cigarettes is bad for us, that's what the mind is for, judging and deciding things.

All the body is doing is trying despeately to carry out the mind's orders.

The problem comes when things change and the

mind wants to issue new orders. Just as Onoda was cut off from all communications with his superiors in the Imperial Japanese Army, for most of us, our body is so disconnected from our mind that there's little or no communication between them.

Your conscious mind — the grown-up, hyper-responsible part of you — can sit around all day long venting about wanting to lose weight. But 999 times out of 1000, your body has no freakin' clue that's what you want. The "war" may have ended decades ago, but since the lines of communication are down your brain's messages about making better eating choices, moving your body more and so on simply aren't getting through.

> *"It's not what you do once in a while,*
> *it's what you do day in and day out that*
> *makes a difference"*
> — Jenny Craig

Disconnection

Once more, many of us are so disconnected from ourselves that there's no longer any meaningful communication between mind and body.

Frequently our idea of trying to make a *change* in our life is to spend time creating fancy propaganda leaflets known as Post-It Notes, which we then affix to the bathroom mirror and refrigerator door to remind ourselves to change...and are shocked and disappointed when they have no impact on our behaviors.

Or, worse, we grab a "gun" and charge directly at that brave Japanese soldier within us in a crazed attempt to defeat it or persuade it to step down!

This works really well in abruptly changing our habits. For one day. Or maybe a week. And then our habit comes roaring back, stronger than ever before.

Because our brave, persistent inner Lt. Onoda who smokes or drinks or eats poorly didn't surrender and didn't commit suicide when we attacked, he just retreated deeper into the jungle until we inevitably turned our attention elsewhere, and then he came back out and continued his mission...of smoking or poor eating or the like.

Trust me, your body eats the wrong foods (and probably in greater quantities than you need to live a vibrant, energetic life) because it genuinely believes it's doing you a good service, that it's helping you enjoy a better life.

Okay, what do we know so far?!

1) Our habits are run by our body

2) Our body is metaphorically lost in the jungles of Lubang island carrying out orders that were given to it long ago

3) For most of us, there's no structure in place to communicate with our own body and *change* its orders (As the famous line from Cool Hand Luke goes: *"What we've got here is a failure to communicate!"*)

You still with me?! We're taking our time with this concept because finally understanding how you really operate from the inside out is fundamental to the changes you've always wanted to make in your life! Instead of recognizing that the underlying problem is a failure to communicate with our own bodies, Big Diet and the glossy monthly magazines subtly (or not so subtly) shift all the blame onto us.

We're told again and again that if we don't reach our health and weight goals it's because we didn't do enough or try hard enough or count enough calories. Of course, you now know that nothing could be further from the truth.

The secret to changing our habits has nothing to do with having more discipline or self-control or will-power!

The secret to changing our habits — whether letting go of negative habits or acquiring positive ones — is no different than the key to any marriage or any relationship.

And that is....

Mutual respect. Honesty. And, especially, *communication*.

> *"Today you are You,*
> *this is truer than true.*
> *There is no one alive*
> *who is Youer than You."*
> — Dr. Seuss

Opening the Lines of Communication

Listen, I enjoy watching the movie *The Secret* and reading about the Law of Attraction as much as anybody.

But I also recognize that these were designed to flatter our minds, to tell the inmates (our thoughts) that they are actually in charge of the asylum (our bodies). The popularity of the movie *The Secret* rests on how it promotes the Supremacy of the Mind and suggests that we really and truly can control our lives by *thinking* differently.

In other words, stuff our Mind *already* believes, and likes hearing from outside sources.

Meanwhile your body keeps soldiering on, trying to help you and serve you as best it can.

We're going to explore in some depth how to repairing the broken, dysfunctional relationship we have with our bodies and finally learn how to communicate with it. This is not meant to be a one-

345

night stand. We're going to go *deep* and rebuild a meaningful relationship with ourselves. Our magnificent bodies have been neglected for far too long. It's time to 'put a ring on it'! Again, let's be super clear on this...

BEING OVERWEIGHT IS NOT YOUR FAULT

Being overweight is the result of several overlapping habits being run by your body, along with a failure of communication by your mind.

Just ahead...in Secret #4 we'll examine the role the mind DOES play in initially acquiring habits and we'll discover how to begin developing positive new habits for ourselves. It's gonna get funner and funner around here!

> *"The world is full of suffering. It is also full of overcoming it."*
> –Helen Keller

SECRET #4:
"You Can't Solve Your Problems by THINKING About Them"

The Inner Workings of Our Brains

Although our habits are run exclusively by our body, they usually get their *start* in our mind. Despite all the good-natured teasing I give to the mind, of course I recognize that it's also a beautiful part of us and deserves understanding. (I mean, we could *all* use a little more understanding, right?!)

So let's take a peek inside our noggins and figure out what we're working with here.

If you stopped the average person on the street and asked her to describe how her brain really worked, she likely wouldn't have the first clue what to tell you. At best she might mention the prevailing "model" of how the mind supposedly works that is popular at the moment.

If she had lived back in Ancient Greece, some 2500 years ago, she would've been taught that the intricacies of our intellect were similar to the ingenious series of aqueducts that carried fresh water from a variety of distant sources into the heart of Athens.

Later, in Victorian times, the brain was compared to the stunningly complex arrangements of hubs (train stations) and pathways (train tracks) that made up the steam railroad network.

In the 1950s, an even more complex network—the telephone system—took over as the metaphor *du jour* about how the brain worked. (By now you should be noticing the pattern...every civilization usually just points to the highest technology of its time as the "best" analogy for the human brain!)

Finally in the 1970s, the still-reigning and perhaps never-to-be-defeated model of the human mind made its debut. According to this latest and greatest analogy, your brain is compared to (what else?!) our highest technology: the *computer*.

According to this metaphor, our brain consists of a RAM—our short-term memory which keeps track of phone numbers and remembers (some of the time!) stuff like where we are driving at the moment.

Meanwhile, a Hard Drive buried deep inside our cerebral cortex or someplace like that supposedly stores our long-term memories and fears and, according to most "experts", is responsible for carrying out our habits.

Under their mechanical model, if we want to change one of our habits—say, eating poorly—then we simply need to change the programming in our RAM (i.e., our daily thoughts) about the outcome we desire...and then that information will somehow be transferred to our internal hard drive and we will soon achieve our desired goal.

If we don't magically succeed in achieving our goal by *thinking* about what we want, then we are commanded to think even harder and more often in order to get there. Wherever there is!

ALICE: "Would you tell me which way I ought to go?"

CHESHIRE CAT: "That depends on where you want to get to."

ALICE: "I don't much care where."

CHESHIRE CAT: "Then it doesn't matter which way you go."

Hold The Presses!

There's only one teeny-tiny, teensy-weensy, itsy-bitsy little problem with this whole mind-as-computer metaphor—it's dead WRONG!

Not only is it wrong, it's not even poetic!

Our brain is a computer? Really?! Nothing else in all of nature is "like" a computer...why should our brains be?!

Seriously, telling people that their brains are computers and can therefore be programmed to make any change they like has probably messed up more people than any other idea or invention in history. (Except perhaps for the invention of the *mirror*, which was no doubt the beginning of our tragic disconnection between mind and body.)

Well here's some breaking news: our brain isn't anything like a computer and it doesn't run on programs like computers do.

As we've already discovered, merely thinking about our habits with the "RAM" of our mind doesn't have any discernible impact whatsoever on our actual habits. Remember, any action or behavior that's been learned well enough to qualify as a habit is now being run by the body, which no longer even looks to the mind for any further instructions or "programming" about the habit.

Just think about it *observationally*. If we COULD consciously program our brains to carry out our wishes the way so many Motivational Speakers encourage us to do, who wouldn't consciously choose to wake up tomorrow on, say, a romantic beach in the Caribbean in the very best shape of our life with millions in the bank and the partner of our dreams right next to us?!

Yet that's not most people's lot in life—even the ones who've watched *The Secret over* and over (and over) again!

In the real world, nobody just *Thinks* and Grows Rich. (They have to think...and *then* do a lot of other stuff with their **body**...and *then* they grow rich!)

Our brains cannot be programmed, only computers can. Some years back I installed PhotoShop on my laptop. I only had to install it the once, and since then anytime I want to run that program I simply open it up and it magically "remembers" how to edit and tweak photographs every single time!

Now if our brains also worked like computers, we'd only have to read *one* self-help book or attend a *single* motivational seminar in our entire life, right?!

Because then we'd be done — our brain would be all re-programmed with the goodness our mind learned and we'd be living our dreams from then on!

For that matter, if it were actually true that all we needed to do was consciously choose to lose weight and our minds would instantly be reprogrammed like installing PhotoShop, then you and I wouldn't even need to be having this conversation right now, would we?! Because you'd already be at your natural weight, in fantastic health, bursting with energy and vitality, and all sorts of other goodness!

I honestly don't think the motivational "experts" and diet gurus are deliberately lying to us when they spend an entire week-end seminar explaining how to use our "computer brain" to reprogram our lives. They're just telling us what other people told them and hoping it actually works this time around. Besides, it's far easier to *market* seminars and products that tout the supremacy of our mind, since it already thinks it's in charge of everything we do and it's the part of us that ultimately makes our purchasing decisions, lulz! So if our brain doesn't work like a Cray supercomputer, how the hell does it operate?

Iceberg Dead Ahead!

There is another popular analogy often used to describe our brains. It's not only much lower-tech and much closer to the truth, but it's also infinitely more poetic.

I'm referring, of course, to the metaphor that compares our mind to an iceberg—those unique, beautiful crystalline structures of frozen water that float majestically on the coldest of seas.

The bright, shiny bits sticking up above the surface of the ocean can be compared to our conscious mind—our immediate thoughts and activities concerning the business of the day. Meanwhile, the vast, dark bulk of the iceberg submerged beneath the waves is considered to be "everything else".

And that's much closer to the way things actually work within us.

Our minds are very much like the small fraction of the iceberg sticking out above the water. Our brains are the only part of us exposed to the "reality" of the outside world. And since it's the only part of us that's more or less visible above the surface we often mistake the mind for the whole iceberg.

Meanwhile, the vast submerged portion of the iceberg is like our *body*, which has no direct exposure to the Reality above the waves, but instead inhabits a dark, beautiful, silent, mysterious world of its own.

Your mind is responsible for interacting with the work-a-day world around you—going to a job, paying bills and other important, grown-up stuff!

Beneath the waves, your body has nothing to contribute to grown-up tasks like paying bills and such. Indeed, your body doesn't have any concept whatsover of what bills are or why you should be paying them in the first place!

Hitting the Snooze Button

Your mind is the part of you that reluctantly drags you out of bed each morning to go to work...because your mind has been told again and again (by other people's minds, for sure!) that hard work is the only path to succeed!

Meanwhile, your body is the part of you tugging at your leg, begging you to call in pretending to be sick so you can spend the day doing something your body loves to do...like playing!

That's not to say your body doesn't work hard. Indeed, as we'll discover, your body works many orders of magnitude harder than your brain...in no small part by running all of your habits, as well as every other complex function that keeps you alive from moment to moment. Yet even though your body runs all your many habits day and night, it doesn't view that as work at all, but rather as games it gets to play.

For many Americans eating poorly is a deeply ingrained habit. So is not moving our body. And so is not loving ourselves.

Again, our habits usually start off as conscious, purposeful actions we take in the world. Most smokers quite deliberately smoked their very first cigarette.

Once the body gets the *message* that any particular action (driving to our new job, biting our nails, drinking the pain away) is important to us, it takes over the action from the mind and repeats it indefinitely without any need for further input or guidance. Again, the key phrase being: "repeats indefinitely".

> *"The essence of education is the education of the body"*
> — Benjamin Disraeli

The Body IS The Show

It's not so much that your body *can* repeat a habit indefinitely, it's that it absolutely WILL repeat it from now on without ever stopping as long as your body continues to believe that it has orders to do so.

This is why some smokers continue puffing away even after they've been diagnosed with cancer.

The body doesn't "think" in terms of good or bad, right or wrong, fat or skinny. That's what the mind is for — *thinking* about things. The body is for *doing* things.

But the conventions of our society, as well as generations of self-help books and motivational gurus, keep insisting that the mind is in charge...of everything!

And so most of humanity walk around pretending the mind is the Big Boss of us, even though we *all* know that most definitely is not true.

After all, many of us spend years and years of our life *thinking* about our problems, but that didn't make a single one of them go away, did it?! If anything, *thinking* about our problems often just makes them worse!

Can I get an Amen?!

> *"Life isn't about finding yourself. Life is about creating yourself."*
> —George Bernard Shaw

The Emperor's Clothes

Yet we're supposed to remain quiet and not speak about any of this out loud. Or at least not loud enough for our brains to overhear the heresy that it's not in charge of everything!

The real tragedy with the prevailing computer analogy of our brains is that it reinforces the false sense of "control" over our lives that we have bestowed upon our minds.

Then when we don't get the results we expected after "reprogramming" our brains for success, we start getting angry at ourselves and look for something within us to blame.

And since it can't be the mind's fault, we blame — what else?! — our innocent body! And because our body doesn't a "voice", it can't easily fight back. Our body silently has to take the fall again and again whenever our lives aren't working out the way we planned.

It has become a time-honored tradition to place the blame for our transgressions on our "flesh" and to punish it in some way, shape or form.

If you'd lived in the Middle Ages, you might have whipped your own back with nail-studded strips of leather whenever you'd been particularly naughty. Nowadays, we punish ourselves by filling up on fat-producing, carbohydrate-laden foods and refusing to let our bodies out to play.

Since virtually our entire culture is built around informing and entertaining the mind and ignoring (at best) the body, nobody is supposed to actually speak up and point out that the Emperor has no clothes.

Our minds get all our free-time, our attention, our entertainment and our praise...while the body gets the table scraps off the Dollar Menu.

We've created an upside-down world where we're almost *forced* to become isolated and divided from ourselves by living through our minds and mistreating our bodies.

And, ohhhhh, how the ugly Stepsisters of the Brain love lording it over the Cinderella of our body!

Then we buy pills and potions and patches in a desperate and doomed attempt to control our body from the outside in.

We spend 100% of our free time engaging and entertaining our brains, then we're absolutely bewildered when our bodies get sick and, ultimately, fall apart totally. We criticize our bodies because criticizing our mind is not permitted!

If you really want to lose weight, sooner or later you're going to have to learn how to:

Get Out of Your Head…And Into Your Body!

"We can begin to heal our lives at the deepest levels when we begin to value our bodies and honor their messages instead of feeling victimized by them."
— Christine Northrup

The Inner Conflict

If you've ever been around someone trying to quit smoking through will-power alone (that is to say, using their "all-great and all-powerful" Oz-brain), it's never a pretty sight. They usually suffer! They usually suffer a lot!

Now they think (oh, how they think!) that they're fighting a battle with cigarettes or something *outside* themselves. And if they can just "put their mind to it" then they'll be able to win the battle with that evil stuff out there.

What they don't realize is that the battle is on the *INSIDE*. Trying to change a negative habit creates an *internal conflict* between their body and their mind.

And, frankly, it's not a fair fight.

The body has so many more resources and so much more capability and power compared to the mind that trying to make lasting changes in our life using our brain alone is like paddling out into the ocean in a rowboat to attack a nuclear-powered aircraft carrier.

That's why barely 4 out of every 100 smokers finally succeed at quitting smoking through will-power alone—that, is by using just their mind. (And, even then, it takes that meager 4% of smokers an average of 6 separate "quit attempts" spread out over a decade to ultimately succeed!)

The real tragedy is that all this time the body was completely unaware there was even a battle going on up above the surface!

In the same way that Lt. Onoda was unaware that World War II had ended, our body has no way of knowing the new orders our mental headquarters comes up with on a near daily basis.

> *"The soul always knows what to do*
> *to heal itself. The challenge is to*
> *silence the mind."*
> —Caroline Myss

Why Dieting Doesn't Work

Suppose I was in the habit of eating what I refer to as Krap on a regular basis. Then one day my friend Abby and I are having coffee and we decide to go on the latest fad diet thingie. Abby and I even shake hands on it. We're serious about dropping the excess weight this time around.

Here's the rub: the part of us that's in charge of losing the weight wasn't even *present* at our little coffee klatsch. I mean, our body was there, physically, but it was doing other stuff and not paying attention to our conversation.

Still, I'm determined to go on my new and I immediately start eating better...or, at least, differently.

A day of good eating passes. Maybe even two or three. But eventually my body is gonna send me a little message. It could be in the form of a tingling on my tongue or a rumbling in my stomach or some other *physical* sensation—*because physical sensations is language the body speaks.*

And the message goes like this, "Hey, Big Spender, let's buy some nice, carb-alicious Krap that we can microwave and scarf down during the 11.5 minutes we have free for lunch today!"

Now my body isn't trying to *sabotage* my dieting efforts...it's completely unaware I'm even on a diet.

My fantastic, loyal and oh so dedicated body is simply repeating its ingrained behavioral pattern—the habit of eating and drinking Krap on a regular basis. Yet the Body would also be perfectly happy to change to a completely different habit once it got the message and understood the new behavior we desired.

The Start of A Beautiful Friendship

I'm not big on homework assignments, as you've probably noticed by now, but I do want to give you one here. At some point in time TODAY I would like you to take the first baby-step in reconnecting with your lovely body.

Your homework is to *spend 15 minutes with your body.*

You can DO anything you want with your body—walk around, climb a tree, skip, or my favorite, dancing.

The only restriction is that you cannot also entertain your mind while you're spending time with your body. (I mean, duh—but it still needs to be said!) That means no listening to music, no watching the news and no doing *anything* other than spending a quarter of an hour in a purely physical realm with your body.

And while you're doing that, be open. *Listen* to your body...whatever that means to you.

Your body gets so few opportunities to

communicate with you and most of those take the form of pain because that's one of the very few ways it can ever override the outside world and actually get your damn attention for a couple of moments.

Right about now your mind might be thinking, quite loudly, "Seriously, 15 minutes of doing nothing?! What a waste of time that would be!"

I'm here to tell you that spending a quarter of an hour with your body is not a waste of time.

Indeed, I'd like to argue that it's *the very best use of your time possible.*

Let's not lose sight of the point of all this. One of the primary goals of the entire *Low Carb Revolution* system is to take you from the weight you are now to your Ideal Body.

Everything I'm sharing with you, and the few homework assignments I'll suggest, are necessary steps on that journey.

This life-changing voyage we've undertaken together will ultimately put your mind and your body back in communication with one another. And that will lead directly to you falling in love with your amazing body for perhaps the first time since you were a child. When we reach that point, making changes in what you eat and how often you play are going to seem like the best idea ever. You'll feel like a giddy newlywed — a groom with the most beautiful bride in history. And what makes a groom happier than anything?! Why, making his *bride* happy, of course! Pampering her and loving her and doting on her.

When your mind becomes a love-struck groom who adores the amazing bride of your body, *that* will be the start of the most beautiful friendship in the history of your life! Okay, let's keep playing!

Coming up next…in Secret #5 we'll learn that our brains *do* play an important role in our ultimate success in losing weight—even if that role is often just staying the hell out of our way so we can succeed!

"The next time you feel like complaining, remember that your garbage disposal probably eats better than 30% of the people in the world"
—Robert Orben

SECRET #5:
"Whether You Think You CAN Lose Weight,
or Think You CAN'T—You're Right!"

The Glass is Half-Full

During WWII, Army doctors and nurses noticed an interesting phenomenon among a certain group of wounded Allied soldiers. These particular soldiers had been grievously injured. Many had lost arms or legs, yet none of their wounds were fatal. In other words, no matter how badly hurt they had been, these troops were expected to live.

Here's the surprising part: these badly wounded soldiers reported less pain and requested less pain medication than soldiers who were only slightly injured.

Even more shockingly, the *morale* of these badly wounded men was higher than both mildly injured soldiers AND soldiers who hadn't been injured at all!

At first the Army medical staff was baffled. How could these soldiers be so upbeat when the war had dealt them such a seemingly cruel hand? After scratching the surface, the doctors and nurses discovered that, despite their injuries, these solders perceived two wins from their situation. First and foremost, they weren't dead! Which, during a time of war, had been a daily, even hourly, possibility up until then. Second, they weren't going to die! Well, at least not in the war, since the gravity of their injuries meant they'd be sent home and would never have to return to the battlefield.

No Man Is An Island

Nothing happens to us in isolation. On the one hand, being physically injured is pretty much universally considered to be a negative experience. On the other hand, if being physically injured ultimately saves our life, then we could say it has a definite upside.

"Bad news" isn't always quite as bad as we first imagine. Indeed, bad news very often turns out to be good news in disguise.

Yes, those soldiers were in bad shape, but an unexpected consequence of their injuries was that they were going to survive the war! Rather than frame their war experience as negative (and who would blame them if they did, what with their terrible injuries?), these brave men chose to frame it in terms of the positive experience of going home.

Our minds fundamentally construct the reality we perceive around us every single moment and it can "spin" that reality in any way that seems appropriate. As our needs and circumstances change, our "reality" can and does change as well.

> *"We are disturbed not by what happens to us, but by our thoughts about what happens to us."*
> —Epictetus

The Thought Virus

Last year my friend Mandy went to a chiropractor because she had some aches and pains following a nasty bicycle crash.

The chiropractor took X-Rays of her hips, then put the film up on the lightbox to examine it. After observing my friend's messed up pelvis for a moment, the chiropractor casually commented, "Wow, you might never be able to have children now!"

Mandy looked at her chiropractor, utterly horrified, wondering why in the world he would tell her something like that.

Without saying a word, she got up and walked the chiropractor's office, never to return. Mandy didn't believe his flip diagnosis. More to the point, she didn't *want* to believe that she could no longer have children. Nor could she imagine any possible benefit to believing that. After a hastily scheduled examination by a real doctor, Mandy ascertained that her womanly parts were just fine and motherhood was still a real possibility for her. (Finding Mr. Right, well, that's another matter!)

The chiropractor had attempted to plant a Thought Virus in her mind…which Mandy fortunately managed to weed out before it ever took root.

The chiropractor's reckless comment wasn't True. Not only that, it also wasn't remotely Useful.

> *"The mind is its own place, and in itself can make a heaven of Hell, a hell of Heaven"*
> —John Milton

"True" versus "Useful"

Letting go of excess weight isn't just about changing some of our negative habits — those activities our body has been doing on auto-pilot without any need to think about them.

It's also a wonderful opportunity for us to create new and empowering habits, both large and small, that will bring us closer to the life we desire and deserve.

One habit I would encourage you to cultivate—deliberately at first, until it becomes, well, a habit!—is to practice framing the stories you tell yourself in terms of whether they are "True" or "Useful".

Bottom line, your REALITY is what you make of it. Both figuratively and literally. You color your perception of everything that happens to you through the filters of your own beliefs and expectations. These "frames" guide our decisions in life and our understandings of how the world around us works. Naturally, certain beliefs and expectations are more useful to us in generating successful outcomes than others, regardless of whether these beliefs are technically "true" or not!

The best example is people who are optimistic. Optimists possess an especially *distorted* view of their own reality. Optimists tend to believe they have more potential, more ability and enjoy more positive outcomes than they "actually" do. Optimists also regularly do silly things like underestimate their pain levels and overestimate their happiness. As you would expect, with Pessimists the reverse is true and according to the frame they see the world through, everything that can possibly go wrong in their life is certain to go wrong sooner or later…if not sooner AND later!

Crazily enough, the harsher grades that Pessimists give themselves on what their life is like are in reality closer to the "truth"!

Yet it's the Optimists who report enjoying better health, and greater financial and romantic fulfillment than those with a firmer grasp of the real world.

I can say with some certainty that somewhere (or perhaps several somewheres!) in the *Low Carb Revolution* I'm introduced an idea or concept that your mind rejected and firmly believed could not possibly be "true".

Even if I backed up the statement with science and support from medical doctors and testimonials and observations from others just like yourself, still your mind might NOT want to believe it to be true or possible.

Here's a strategy I'd like to offer to you...

When you come to those moments, both in this book and elsewhere in your life, consider putting aside your brain's initial judgment about whether something is true or false (whatever that even means!) and ask yourself instead, "Is this *useful* to me?"

> *"There is nothing either good or*
> *bad, but thinking makes it so"*
> —William Shakespeare, *Hamlet*

The "Addictive-Free" Cigarettes

The actor Jason Beghe underscores the difference between "true" and "useful" in a compelling story about one of his attempts to quit smoking cigarettes. Beghe had heard that one effective strategy for stopping is to switch to a different brand of cigarettes, which, in theory (and, I hasten to add, *only* in theory; this is neither a "true" nor a "useful" method to help you quit smoking!) you will supposedly find so unpalatable or something that you will magically be done with cigarettes forever.

In Jason Beghe's case, the brand he switched to was a natural blend called American Spirits. He was drawn to them because of the bold assertion printed right on the front of the pack: "Addictive Free!"

Well, that was just the kind of cigarettes Beghe wanted, the kind that weren't *addictive*!

In short order, he cut back from his two-pack per day habit all the way down to merely one cigarette per day! And since they weren't addictive, his next step was to cut out that final, solitary cigarette and join the lovely family of non-smokers.

There was just one little hitch. Just before Jason Beghe meant to stop smoking his last, lone daily cigarette, he shared his success story with a friend. His friend (who, like most people, cared much more about True than Useful) pointed out that Jason been *misreading* the label of his American Spirits all this time.

The front of the box, the "friend" helpfully pointed out, actually read, "Additive-Free", NOT, "Addictive-Free"!

Of course, this little piece of information was demonstrably True...and so in short order Jason Beghe found himself once again smoking his customary two packs per day.

It was True...but not remotely Useful.

> *"To be a great champion you must*
> *believe you are the best. If you're*
> *not, pretend you are."*
> —Muhammad Ali

In a Quantum World Nothing is True

In my estimation, the greatest self-help book of all time remains Dale Carnegie's classic, *How to Win Friends and Influence People.*

In his lively, still-readable book, Carnegie explores this same concept of "True" versus "Useful" (although he calls it something different, of course) across the span of several chapters. He gives repeated examples about how the surest way to NOT win friends is to walk around trying to be Right about everything all the time.

And in the quantum world we live in, who's to say what reality is anyway?! If you ask the real experts,

Quantum Physicists, they will answer that the "truth" is that there is nothing anywhere...there is only the *potential* for something to be there.

Again, true, but not particularly useful when I'm trying to walk through a closed door.

I like learning things (no big surprise there, huh?!) and I'm a bit of a documentary junkie. One day not too long ago I stumbled upon a full-length, online documentary called, *Did Jesus Really Exist?* or something along those lines. I decided to check it out. So I start watching this documentary and it was very well-produced, very cleverly put together and narrated, and it made a fairly compelling case that the historical figure known as Jesus never actually existed.

Then, suddenly—I was like maybe 20-25 minutes into the documentary, I hit PAUSE and I asked myself the following question..."Suppose this documentary *has* assembled an airtight case and it is, in fact, 'true' that the historical person we know as Jesus never existed, what possible 'use' would that be in my life?!"

And I had to answer, "Absolutely none at all."

Now I had a classic Catholic upbringing and attended Catholic school all the way up until the day I matriculated into the University of Texas at Austin to complete my formal education. I remain spiritual to this day, but I wouldn't consider myself particularly "churchy". Even so, I'm down with Jesus! He was the Man! And I certainly don't wanna believe he didn't exist. One of the most loving, caring, forgiving persons in the history of the world never really lived?! Sorry, we all need our Heroes...and Jesus is certainly one of mine.

So I stopped watching the documentary and have no particular intention to ever go back and finish watching it, because I'm far less concerned these days with what's "real" than what is "useful" for taking my life to the next level.

Try it for yourself and discover how it feels. Ask yourself now and again, "Whether or not this is *true*, is it useful for me to know or do?" And if it is, keep knowing it or doing it!

Wow, I just wanted to stop and take a moment to tell you that you're doing a great job here! I'm really proud of you for sticking with this, for taking the time out of your schedule to keep reading the *Low Carb Revolution* and consider an entirely new way of thinking about yourself, your mind and your body — and how they can work together to help you lose weight without the inner conflict or turmoil or pain of other methods you may have tried in the past.

When we get to the point where we are seriously *Overwheat* (lulz!) then we are often hiding.

Hiding from ourselves...and the world...behind an excess of body mass that believes it's protecting and cocooning us.

As we continue to go down this road, we'll continue the all-important process of Waking Up! Many of us have been on auto-pilot, letting our habits run us for a long, long time. But now we're waking up and rediscovering ourselves and who we really are and why we're here.

This is exciting stuff. We're on an exciting journey together. So let's keep going, shall we?!

> *"I don't like myself, I'm crazy about myself!"* — Mae West

SECRET #6:
"The Story of Your Problem IS the Problem!"

There's a Bear in Them There Woods

Imagine you're out in the woods and suddenly you see a bear. So you start running—and you hope to God it's the kind of bear you're supposed to run from and not the sort of bear you're supposed to fall down and not move! Now pretend that I came running up alongside you and asked *why* you were running.

You'd probably say something to the effect of, "Dude, I saw this bear and I realized the only way to save my life is to run like crazy, so I made a decision to start running and here I am!"

Okay, that sounds plausible enough. But...is that what REALLY happened?! Is that true? I'm going to suggest to you that, in fact, that's *not* what happened. That's just a "story" you're telling about what happened.

Like so many of the things we think we know, the truth is the exact opposite of what we believe! And the truth is...we always have a story! But the story comes SECOND, not first! Stick with me here, this is gonna get good!

What's the Story Here?

What the hell do I mean by this? I mean that during all our waking hours we constantly feel sensations in our body and we move our body through space to a greater or lesser degree. Our mind is perched there atop our body, pretty much just along for the ride, and it usually has very little to do when it comes to the functioning of our body.

So, to pass the time, our brain LOVES to come up with stories. Listening to and telling stories is our brain's absolute most favorite thing in the world — always has been, always will be.

Whenever *anything* happens to us, no matter how inconsequential, we tell ourselves a *story* about what happened.

The stories we tell ourselves are just our brain's way of *spinning* whatever is going on with our body so it makes sense to our mind. By the bye, we typically believe the stories we tell ourselves to be "true" even when we also know damn well the story is not remotely "useful" for any of the outcomes we desire in our life!

To really understand this, let's return to our account above, the one in where you're running in the woods and I come up to ask why.

Regardless of your answer, here's what REALLY happened, from a scientific perspective...

1) Your legs started moving very quickly beneath you

2) Your digestion (and other "trivial" body systems) immediately shut down

3) You experienced vaso-constriction — with valuable blood flowing away from your skin (and your neo-cortex, the most "thinky" part of your brain) and toward your vital organs in the interior of your body

4) Your reptile brain took over in an effort to help you survive whatever you're experiencing

5) Your amygdala fired and put you into full-on

Fight-or-Flight response.

6) Adrenaline and a host of related "stress hormones" flooded your system, giving you peak energy and responsiveness in the threat of a life-or-death danger

Only AFTER all that takes place does your Brain finally kick in and try to put some *meaning* on your experience.

It desperately wants to create a *story* to explain why you are running full-tilt through the woods. So your brain rewinds the "surveillance tapes" it's constantly recording through your High-Def Eyeball Cameras, and it doesn't have to rewind much before it discovers something really interesting: a Bear!

And that's all your mind needs to create your current story...you saw a bear in the woods and so you started running. Case closed. *Quod erat demonstrandum.*

> *"You, yourself, as much as*
> *anybody in the entire universe,*
> *deserve your love and affection"*
> —Buddha

Split-Brains

Now, in this particular case, the "story" actually happened to be true—in the sense that there really *was* a bear in the woods.

As often as not, however, there's no bear at all. We're running as fast as we can to escape from something that's not even there.

Big Diet usually tells us a story that we are overweight because we overate too many calories...a story that is neither true nor useful.

In fact, as we discovered in Part One, the exact opposite is the truth. We overeat *because* we are overweight. The physiological forces and hormones running rampant in our body when we become obese causes an increase in hunger and requires a greater consumption of food than when we weigh less. And when we eat the wrong types of food (especially the "diet" foods sold to us so relentlessly by Big Diet/Big Food), we become more overweight, which causes us to overeat more—and no wonder that for the first time in history they are now having to make scales that go to 400 pounds for both medical facilities and home use!

We are never without our stories *because they are what allow us to understand our environment and our place within it on an ongoing basis.*

The corpus collosum is the Habi-trail that connects the left and right hemispheres of our brain. As a general rule, we process visual images on one side of our brain and speech on the other.

It sometimes happens (to treat severe epileptic seizures, for example) that people have their corpus collosum completely severed. They are subsequently referred to as split-brain patients—because the two halves of their brain are literally split apart and can no longer communicate with one another. (Not unlike, say, most people's mind and their body, wouldn't you say?!)

Because of their condition, split brain patients' visual and speaking centers are not connected, and researchers have fashioned some interesting experiments for them.

Now these people are unable to describe something they are looking at with spoken words, since the part of their mind that is *seeing* has no physical contact with the part of the brain that processes *speech*.

In one classic experiment, they showed split-brain patients a series of clever New Yorker cartoons.

The split-brain patients would process the cartoon

371

and then laugh out loud. But here's where it really got interesting. They were then asked to tell the researchers WHY they were laughing.

Keep in mind, these people have NO way of actually telling the researchers *why* they were laughing since their hemispheres were not *physically connected* to one another.

So what do you think happened? Do you think the patients said, "Hey, I have no idea why I'm laughing!" or, "I can't say!" Well, no. *We always have a story, remember?!*

And these patients always had an answer. The split-brain patients would say something like, "Oh, I laughed because I just recalled that one time I caught a cab outside the United Nations building and the cabbie said the funniest thing!"...basically the kinds of completely outlandish fabrications that teenagers tell to teachers and parents and seriously expect them to believe.

So the *story* the split-brain patients told about why they were laughing had literally nothing to do with reality (i.e., the cartoon they were looking at) yet that was their story and they were sticking to it!

We Are All Healers

After pulling myself out of the chain-smoking, overweight, broke-ass bitch hole I had dug for myself during many long years of personal neglect, I began working with others to help turn their lives around. Smoking-cessation and weight-loss were the obvious places to start testing my revolutionary new theories.

Success followed success, and over time I discovered some ancient yet highly effective methods to help people let go of the most serious traumas in their life.

Before long I was working with private clients

across the entire spectrum of "problems" that people have in this day and age.

Besides achieving many profound victories in helping people to help themselves, I also uncovered a general principle that changed the way I understood the entire healing process.

I personally believe that we are all natural Healers. Only a few us decide to identify as Healers—in the same way that only a few of us decide to identify as being Creative or Entrepreneurial, etc.—but we all have the ability to heal ourselves and to help others heal. Again, that's my considered belief. Now, should you one day decide to let your own inner Healer out to play and work with people who need, well, healing, what you'll quickly (i.e., immediately!) discover is that everybody has a *story* about their "problem".

"All healing is self-healing"
— Albert Schweitzer

We've *All* Got A Story

And the story of our problem can be quite the story! It can have all the twists and turns and set-backs of a Greek tragedy. If we've had the problem long enough then the story may well grow to epic proportions. And many of us *love* telling the story of our problem, whatever it may be.

One day I was working with someone who had just launched into telling me "the story of her problem", and I had an epiphany. Two of them, in fact.

Epiphany the First: The "problem" she described in her story about it wasn't even her actual problem...it was just a collection of *symptoms* caused by her real problem.

Epiphany the Second: *The story we tell ourselves about our problems often IS the problem.*

This second epiphany, especially, was a game-changer for me.

Once I wrapped my mind around the realization that the more we repeat to ourselves and to others a specific story about our problems, the more legitimacy, support and reinforcement we give to that difficulty in our life.

> *"The mind that perceives the*
> *limitation is the limitation"*
> — Buddha

The Story IS the Problem

In a phrase…

The story we tell ourselves about our problem often IS the problem.

How often have you heard members of your Tribe tell and retell negative stories about themselves?

"Oh, I can't learn how to juggle…I'm too clumsy"…"Nobody will ever love me again…I'm too old"…"I am just a smoker and there's nothing I can do about it"…"The pollen count in this city always gives me seasonal allergies"…"I'm overwheat *because my father was a baker and I'm genetically unable to stop eating bread"*

Suppose the story I tell myself is, "I'm overweight and nothing can change that."

As long as I buy into my story about being overweight and not being able to do change that, then I'm going to find a way to keep that story going by doing whatever it takes to not lose weight. Because if I started losing weight, that would totally *ruin* the story I've been telling myself all these years, you see?!

374

In fact, being "permanently overweight" is just a story I've been telling myself.

The truth is I am not overweight. My natural state, my birthright, is to be in my Ideal Body.

Sure, I may currently weigh more than I would like, but that's not who I am, it's just a story I keep telling myself. Often the stories we tell ourselves revolve around what our body is capable or not capable of. We tell ourselves these stories in our heads...yet our brains has absolutely no conception of what our body is actually capable of accomplishing or not.

The main problem with the stories we tell ourselves is that they are a) often not True; b) almost never Useful. When people try to quit smoking cigarettes on their own, after a day or so they may report feeling tired, listless and tense.

So the *story* they tell themselves next goes something like this: "The physical sensation I'm feeling in my body right now means I'm craving a smoke and I will die unless I go smoke a cigarette right now!"

But we've already learned that the physical sensations come *first* and the story comes *second*. What that means is that the story we tell ourselves about the physical sensations (i.e., cravings) in our body can be *any story we want*. Remember, the physical sensations in our body are *real*. The stories we tell ourselves about the *meaning* of those very real physical sensations are often completely made up.

How many times have you had a momentary, sharp pain in your side and your very first thought was, "Oh my God, I must have cancer—that's gotta be a tumor I'm feeling"?! Lord knows I've done that a thousand times, go from an isolated, sharp pain to my own death sentence in the span of a single breath, and then it passes and ten minutes later I've forgotten all about it.

Fear of Public Speaking

It's said that for many Americans public speaking is their #1 fear, that they'd rather die than get up and speak in front of an audience.

Now if you were to interview a person who was terrified of public speaking and they were about to go on stage to give a presentation in front of a big audience, and you asked them what they were *feeling* right now, in their body, they might say something like…

Butterflies in stomach
Tingling in throat
Tightness in shoulders
Uncomfortable surge of energy throughout body

So first they experience all those physical sensations. And only then do they create a story to explain the sensations.

And the story that explains these particular sensations goes like this: "Oh Jeez, I'm terrified! I'm gonna die here! This is awful. I feel terrible! I can't talk in front of these people!"

Do you get the distinction here? It's NOT that they have a fear of public speaking and that fear causes certain body sensations to remind them how afraid they are. It IS that they experience certain body sensations and *then* their mind tells a story about the meaning of those sensations.

What we were taught…

Story -> Physical Sensations in Body

What really happens…

Physical Sensations in Body -> Story

Love of Public Speaking

Let me share with an example of how changing the story we tell ourselves about our "problem" can make all the difference in the world.

Some years ago I had the privilege of working for the legendary author, speaker and life coach, Tony Robbins. You know, the "big teeth" guy!

I was one of his Sales Trainers in the field and also worked with him directly on those days when he presented seminars to many thousands of people. I've been backstage with Tony Robbins before a big seminar. I can assure the sensations he felt in his body were similar, if not identical, to the ones in the example above.

Butterflies in stomach
Tingling in throat
Tightness in shoulders
Exhilerating surge of energy throughout body

In other words, Tony Robbins probably feels 99.9% of the *exact same bodily sensations* as people who are utterly terrified of public speaking.

The only difference is the story Tony Robbins tells himself before he goes on stage. And here's what Tony Robbins is probably thinking in his head, here's the story he's telling himself about the meaning of those same exact physical sensations in his body...

"I'm so excited right now because I have an opportunity to connect with this amazing group of people I've never met before. They spent good money to be here and I might have only this one chance to influence them and inspire them and give them value, so I really hope I can help them and maybe send them home with some tools or strategies that will make a lasting difference in their life!"

Same planet, different worlds.

When we feel physical sensations in our body, we almost always have a wide degree of latitude about deciding what they mean, in other words, what story we're going to put on them.

I mean, we already do this all the time...almost randomly assign stories to the sensations we experience!

Fear of Hiccups

Every single day of our lives we feel numerous physical sensations in our body. With the familiar sensations (stomach growling) we automatically assign a story (I'm hungry) and then seek a resolution (the Old You: McTacoHut...the New You: Food!).

With unfamiliar sensations, though, oftimes our first impulse is to freak the hell out! We decide the slightest unusual pain in our neck is the portent of a quick and horrendous death (or a slow and painful death...or, when we're really on a roll, *both*!) Even when the unusual physical sensation has dissipated a short time later, the grim story we told ourselves about it sort of still lingers in the air.

A classic example of getting caught up in our own story comes whenever we get the Hiccups.

When you think about it, the hiccups themselves are no big deal. You're taking an extra gulp of air a couple of times a minute is all. They don't hurt or anything. But what happens when we get the hiccups? We PANIC and freak out!

"OMG, I've got the *hiccups*! I'm never gonna get rid of them! I'm gonna be like that girl in Florida who had hiccups for 4 years! Ahhhhhhhh!"

The story that most of us put on hiccups is so out of proportion to the actual impact of hiccups — not least since we usually figure out some way to get rid of them within half an hour or less — that the entire experience is completely laughable. Well, except when it's *us* who has the hiccups, right?!

Listen to Your Body

As you continue the process of reconnecting with your body and rebuilding its relationship with your mind, I'd like for you to become more, shall we say, "open", to interpreting the signals your body is sending to you. In the West especially we tend to move in the opposite direction *away* from particularly strong sensations in our body — whether pleasurable or painful.

Back when I a chain-smoking, overweight couch potato, I got headaches literally 7 days per week. At the first glimmer of a headache I would gulp down two Ibuprofen. I usually had the "first glimmer of a headache" every 6 hours, which is the minimum allowable time between doses of Ibuprofen, go figure! As I began the journey of Transformation that led me to where I am today, at a certain point I realized that maybe my body was trying to tell me something...and *that* was the reason for the chronic headaches in the first place.

So the next time I felt the tell-tale onset of a headache, I stopped. I didn't reach for the Ibuprofen. Instead I directed my attention inward, towards the pain itself. And I listened. I just sat there quietly for a few moments, open to any communication from my body.

Now my body didn't actually say anything to me. The body doesn't speak words, of course. It didn't say, "Hey, Johnny Boy, now that I've got your attention, please eat more green beans" or anything like that.

But it *did* say something on some level and I listened in whatever way I knew how. After that my body seemed happy and the pain in my head went away.

On those rare times now when I feel the twinges of a

mild headache coming on, I tell myself a completely new story. Recall that the old story was that I needed to hurriedly take some pills to make the pain go away.

The new story is that my body is probably trying to communicate with me somehow and it would be a capital idea for me to stop what I'm doing and spent a few moments listening to it!

> *"If you want to hold the beautiful one, hold*
> *yourself to yourself"*
> —Rumi

Eeeeeek, Another Homework Assignment!

For your homework assignment this time around I would love for you to continue growing the relationship and rekindling the romance between your body and mind. To do that, I want you to start listening to your body when its communicating to you through physical sensation—whether pain or pleasure.

That means turning toward the sensations in your body rather than away from them.

You can always reach for your version of "Ibuprofen" later. If possible, first spend a few minutes listening to what your body is trying to communicate to you.

The magic of this is that your body *knows* when you are listening. The very first time you stop and devote your undivided attention to "listening" to a new or unusual physical sensation in your body, your incredible body may well be utterly dumbfounded and shocked by the attention your paying it. But keep doing it and the rewards will be great.

Listen, if your body knows you're listening to it, then that also opens a channel of communication where it will start listening to you.

Communication can and should be a two-way

street. Listen to your body AND be aware that you might benefit from telling yourself a completely different story about what you're experiencing in your body!

Just ahead in Secret #7, we're going to explore a radically obvious step in our journey to lose weight that has been totally overlooked by every single one of the "Diet gurus".

> *"Become more aware of how you choose to*
> *treat this miracle of a body. Talk to it as you*
> *give it exercise, good food and generous*
> *amounts of fresh water."*
> —Dr. Wayne Dyer

SECRET #7:
"You Are Not Who You Think You Are"

The Most Important-est Secret of Them All

Now I recognize that I'm Captain Superlative. Everything with me is always the "most" this and the "best" that and I've apparently never met an exclamation point I didn't like! So when I start things off in this chapter by referring to it as "the most important-est Secret of them all" I realize you might want to take that with a grain of salt...or three.

Even so, I strongly believe this particular secret will introduce you to a concept of personality and behavior that will change the way you think about yourself and others forever.

The personality model called Parts Theory we're about to explore in this chapter and the next is not well known outside the world of personal counseling and therapy. (And even in *that* world it's not widely known!)

Yet this profound model can be applied directly to changing our habits — both good and bad — as well as to transforming any aspect of our personal, professional and romantic lives.

The radical concept of Parts Theory you're about to discover is likely to be *completely different* from anything you've ever been exposed to before...and that's why I've come along to share it with you!

If you're gonna color, you might as well color

outside the lines, right?!

At the same time, as you begin to understand this model I suspect you will increasingly find parallels in your own life and behaviors...until before long you'll be able to point to several different parts within *yourself* who are responsible for many of the otherwise unexplainable decisions "you" have made in the past!

Who Are You, Anyway?!

Let's jump right into this with a truth you may not have considered before. You are not who other people think you are, are you?! The rest of the world sees you as a single, monolithic entity with a name and a label.

You're Sally...the pastor's wife
You're Cedric...an acting coach
You're Maureen...a student
You're Gretchen...a politician
You're Waldo...and nobody can find you, lulz!

And so on. But you're not just any *one* of the things you do in your life—athlete, daughter, academic, survivor, mom or artist.

Yes, sometimes you are a mom and the part of you that's a mom comes out and is all "mom-like" and stuff. But when you're out having drinks with your girlfriends, the last thing in the world you want to do is "bring out" the part of you that's a mom! The entire *point* of hanging out with your girlfriends is to give the mom part of you a break and let another part of you out to play!

By the same token, if your romantic partner is coaxing out the sexual side of you one night and suddenly one of your children starts crying from another room, the part of you that's a mom is normally gonna return with a vengeance and you're going to rush to check on your child.

There's a part of you that's creative, a part of you that's sexual, a part of you that's spiritual and so on. And there's only room—or bandwidth, let's call it—for *one* part of us to be out at a time.

"What Did I Come In Here For?!"

Have you ever had this experience…

You're sitting on the sofa watching TV and you remember that you cooked a huge meal the night before and there are still plenty of leftovers in the refrigerator. So you decide it would be a lovely idea to go warm up a nice snack in the microwave. At the next commercial break, you dutifully scramble into the kitchen. And as soon as you get there, you stop dead.

You think, "What the hell did I come in the kitchen for?! I know I came in here to get something but I have no clue what it was. (Let me be the first to reassure you—this *isn't* because you're bonkers or because you're suffering from early onset dementia because you drank away too many brain cells in college or anything of the kind.

It *is* because…the part of you that was sitting there vegging on the couch, watching CSI: Mars or whatever, is literally NOT the same part of you that is all organized and managerial and knows how to get food out of the fridge and microwave it, etc.

These are two completely separate "parts" of you…and they're not very good at talking to one another.)

So what happens?! You stand there dumbly in the kitchen for a moment, still with no recollection of why you walked in there. Reluctantly you return to the living room, and as you do, the "couch-potato" part of you returns and yells, "Tell 'em to take the food out of the refrigerator and heat it up!"

And only *then* does the message finally get through

from one part of you to the other and you can return to the kitchen to complete the task at hand.

We Are Made of Parts

Let's clear up an important mystery right away. Even if you *do* sometimes overeat or binge-eat or any variation on that theme, it's probably not even YOU who's doing it, but rather a *part* of you.

Something they never teach you in school is that we are all made up of various "parts" who take turns doing all the various wonderful (and sometimes not-so-wonderful) things we do.

There's a part of us that knows how to do our day job, a part of us that's spiritual, a part of us that's sexual, a part of us that's entrepreneurial , a part of that can be wildly creative and on and on.

We all have certain parts in common. (As I mentioned earlier, we all have an Inner Healer…whether or not we ever let that part of us out to play is a different story altogether.) And we each have parts that are *unique* to us. Some of us have a part within us that's often hungry or often in pain or often worried…and this is the part of us that usually engages in our wild extremes in eating.

You could almost say this part has a job. And that job is to punish us or reward us or console us or whatever job this part thinks it's supposed to do for us. These parts of us are also often really good at their job. They sometimes never forget to take action.

Like the famous Lt. Onoda, the various parts of us will damn well keep doing their job forever unless and until new orders come along to change them..

If we're going to join the Revolution to return to our Ideal Body, we're also going to have make friends with our parts and then take a rather radical step. And, no, the radical step is not to "get rid" of our offending

385

parts!

Parts Are Here to Stay

All of has several parts in common—Universal parts that do specific "jobs" for each and every one of us. And we all have several (sometimes several dozen) part that are *unique* to us, parts that do jobs large (chainsmoking) and small (knitting once a month) and everything in between.

Whether universal or unique, we cannot get rid of our parts, of course. Once we have a part, we have it forever.

People who smoke cigarettes have an internal "part" of them that smokes the cigarettes. People who drink too much alcohol have a part of them to do that.

Let's cut to the chase: the "overeating part" within you is ALWAYS going to be a part of you. It's always going to have its own unique drive, energy and enthusiasm. It's always going to have a job and it's always going to do its job.

But, here's the big-money chunk: *Its job doesn't have to be the job it currently does!*

The part of us that now smokes, drinks, binges, etc. can *learn* to do something else instead. In fact, a part of us will often gladly sign up for almost any job we desire, it just wants to keep busy and stay productive. Keep in mind, the only reason this part arose and evolved in the first place was because at a certain young age we needed help.

Overeating (or smoking or shoplifting, etc.) was a way to be cool or rebellious or different from others or the same as others...all important needs, especially at an impressionable age.

Our "unique parts" usually arise in an instant to handle a "job" that no other current part can do or, perhaps, wants to do. If you think that our parts are all one big happy family inside of us, you best think again!

Most of our parts exist in *isolation* from the others. A part may be vaguely aware of some of our other parts, but normally they don't communicate or collaborate with one another.

In fact, the prevailing attitude amongst most people's parts is *competitive*.

Think about it, any time you let your Inner Kindergartner out to play for a couple of hours, that necessarily means your Inner Accountant is gonna have to cool her heels until she gets to spend time doing her job, and so on.

When I work with people for Smoking Cessation, I ask them how the part of them responsible for smoking gets along with their ofther parts, and smokers invariably respond, "Oh, the smoking part of me is not popular at all. The other parts really dislike it!"

> *"The world belongs to the energetic"*
> —Ralph Waldo Emerson

The Captain of the Ship

You ever have coffee with a friend and she's asking for your help in making a big decision and she says something like, "Well, a part of me wants to go someplace...but then this other part of me totally doesn't want to go and it wants to do something else instead."

That's what we're talking about here. The various parts that make up who we are each have completely different goals and desires and needs. Returning to a balanced, happy life means giving all the positive, meaningful parts of us a chance to shine!

Now it's not just a free-for-all inside of us, to be sure! We each have an inner Captain of the Ship, if you will, who helps decide which part gets to do its job at any given time.

Our Captain tries to make sure that when we arrive at the office our Inner Worker comes out rather than our Inner S&M Dominatrix. (Well, I guess that depends on where exactly we work, eh?!) If we're the kind of person who goes to Church, well then that's a very good opportunity to spend time with our Spiritual part and it's the Captain who makes that call.

People sometimes say to me, "Wait, there's not like really a little Mini-Me inside me that knows how to play guitar and another that knows how to speak French and another that smokes cigarettes, is there?!"

And I answer: "No, not at all. This is just a *metaphor* to describe how humans universally organize their internal experiences.

But, on the other hand, yes, for all practical purposes it certainly *seems* like there's an actual avatar within us responsible for specific behaviors and actions."

> *"We don't have one mind, we have*
> *competing interests, all duking it out"*
> —Seth Godin

We can better understand how the Parts Model really works by an example of a spectacular "failure" and the subsequent healing of this very system.

It's a true story I call simply…

Sally's Story

Once upon a time a few years ago I had a private client named "Sally", who was a highly driven woman in her late-twenties working for a high-technology company. When Sally came to me, she was, by her own account, "a complete mess".

One day, six months earlier, Sally and a fellow

manager were at work. They turned a corner and caught a low-level employee loafing around on the job one too many times. While Sally watched, her fellow manager summarily fired the loafer, who grumbled under his breath and stormed out.

The next day Sally and her fellow manager were back at work as usual. Suddenly the door opened and the former employee strolled in. Wearing a black trench coat. And carrying a gun.

He strode right up to the other manager and shot him point blank in the face with bullet after bullet, almost completely obliterating his entire head. Meanwhile, in slow-motion, Sally scrambled and dove under a table to take some sort of cover. As the last shell hit the floor, the killer slowly turned and walked directly towards the table where Sally was hiding. He stopped walking and deliberately bent over to look under the table, then smiled weakly at her.

"I would never hurt you, Sally", he said, and strolled out the door like nothing happened. The killer got in his car, drove a few blocks…and then blew his own brains out.

So that's what happened to Sally that day. And who wouldn't be a complete mess after going through such an horrific experience?!

Where Did Sally Go?

When I first met Sally she was suffering from full-blown Post-Traumatic Stress Disorder (PTSD), which all the doctors and all the pills in the world couldn't put back together again.

With my background in hypnosis, NLP, shamanism and other esoteric healing arts, I recognized that I wasn't going to be anybody's "first stop" for healing anything—but it turned I knew exactly how to help Sally.

Her PTSD was so severe that she had to quit her former high-tech job because she was totally unable to return to her old workplace. For that matter, Sally was unable to leave her own house unless one or more friends (one of them was an actual Army MP on leave!) accompanied her. Worst of all, much of her formerly beautiful, curly blonde hair had fallen out in huge clumps...leaving unsightly bald spots on her scalp. This meant she had to don a wig before she could even set foot past her front door.

Equally frustrating, this formerly highly organized, super-industrious alpha-female now found herself scatter-brained, disorganized and only intermittently productive.

Often Sally couldn't even remember the details of how to perform even the simplest of tasks. For example, if dirty dishes were stacking up in the kitchen sink, Sally couldn't simply write down on her To Do List: "Wash dishes". Instead, she had to write herself a note saying, "Put dirty dishes in sink". And another note saying, "Add soap to dish scrubber doo-jobber". Another: "Use scrubber doo-jobber to wash off dishes, then rinse in clear water". And finally, "Put dishes in dish-rack to dry".

She told me that the mirrors in her bedroom and bathroom were covered with dozens and dozens of similar Post-It notes, guiding her through formerly routine tasks. "It's like the *organizer* part of me that knows how to do all these things is no longer there," Sally reported. "Or, if she is there, I can't figure out how to communicate with her anymore!"

"We're Going to Need a Bobcat!"

During our first session, I put Sally into hypnosis and together we explored what was going on beneath the surface of her now stormy life.

390

The intense emotional tragedy of the murder she'd witnessed had led to a "wall" of sorts being built in her mind. Her inner Captain had seemingly been *walled off* from the other parts of her...most likely in order to protect it from any harm.

This is no different than the Secret Service creating a human wall in order to protect the President of the United States during times of direct threat.

So in the exact traumatic moments when the shooting took place, Sally's "Captain" was walled off from the rest of her. In a very real sense, the "Captain" was stuck on one side of the wall, dealing with the ongoing pain of the experience, while her many, disparate parts were on the other, safe from danger, but wandering around aimlessly...aware that the Captain of the Ship had gone away, but with no idea where she went or why.

This metaphorical wall sheltered Sally's psyche during the endless moments it took for the terrible tragedy to play itself out.

But now, months later, the wall was still there, of course. Sally (in the form of her internal "Captain") was on one side of it and the many Parts of her that did all the important jobs for her every day were on the other side.

And *that* was the reason for the notes she had to write herself — because no other internal communication was getting through the Wall within her.

In the past Sally could just remind herself to do her taxes and she'd sit down and the part of her that knew how to do taxes would come "out" and do them. But with her lines of communication severed, none of Sally's parts knew what they were supposed to be doing or when they were supposed to do it.

The entire purpose of our first session was to let

Sally and all her parts know that the danger had passed and that she was now *safe* again. This was something her inner parts did not previously know because, again, they were "cut off" from the rest of her.

Sally's continuing trauma, stress and hair loss were occurring because her internal parts still thought they were in immediate danger from the killer.

At the culmination of the first session, we "gathered together" all the various parts of Sally into a sort of virtual town meeting and she calmed them down and reassured them the mortal danger was now past…and let them know they'd be back in business before long.

Over the course of the next week, Sally reported being much calmer and less stressed out as her previously terrified inner parts began to relax and prepare to get back to work again.

During our second and final session, the goal was to breach the wall separating her Inner Cap'n from her other parts. One of her key parts, which she termed the Organizer, was in charge of this mission. (Her Organizer was sort of like the XO on a naval ship. While the Captain is in charge, for all practical purposes the XO runs the ship and gives the bulk of the orders.)

When confronted with the internal wall that needed to be knocked down, Sally's internal Organizer remarked casually, "We're gonna need a Bobcat!"

Moments later, in Sally's mind, her Organizer came rolling up in Bobcat—one of those small, personal tractor/bulldozer machines—and ploughed right through the metaphorical wall, freeing the Captain and returning normalcy to her mind.

The Captain was at last reunited with all the other parts that made up Sally. They had a little party together and made plans to get back to the beautiful game of being Sally once again.

"What's A Bobcat?"

The first thing Sally said after her second, triumphant session, "What's a Bobcat?"

Although she had no conscious knowledge of a Bobcat bulldozer was, the take-charge part of her helping from the other side of the wall surely did.

Sally made a spectacular recovery after only two sessions of working together. She recovered her ability to get things done, and found a new job. Her beautiful, curly blonde hair grew back and she was able to come and go from her house with ease.

In fact, I ran into her only 3 months after our final session and she told me she had just returned from a weekend-long camping trip in the woods—all alone! I was impressed with her, to say the least!

The Parts Model

Now there are many roads to Rome and this is just one of them. In my experience, I have found that the Parts Model helps us make sense of our lives and decisions not only when we are "sick" and need healing, but also in business, social and sexual situations.

We're taking a fair bit of time here together to explore the concept that we are made up of various Parts who take turns being a student, a parent, a clown or whatever because most people have never, ever been exposed to this model of human personalities before.

As with many of the other lessons I've been sharing with you, once you really grasp the Parts Model it will throw open the doors to an amazing new understanding of yourself and *why* you do the things you do.

If you've ever felt you couldn't "help yourself" from overeating or indulging in the wrong types of foods, now you realize that it wasn't even YOU who was doing this, but just one little dedicated (if misguided) part of you.

The Parts Model I've just shared with you also neatly explains why, when faced with decisions, we all often reach the point where one part of us wants to do X and another part wants to do Y! Well, of course, they do!

In exactly the same way that in a large family each of the kids will have a different idea of where they want to go for their summer vacation, each of our parts has different goals and different contributions to make to the adventure of being who we are.

"Why'd You Do That?!"

Our whole lives, whenever we get in trouble, grown-ups always want to know, "Why did you do that?!" Whether the "grown-up" in question is a 3rd grade teacher, our current boss, a jilted lover or Officer Krupke—they all want to know *why* we did whatever bad or stupid thing we did.

But here's the rub: By the time we get caught doing whatever we were doing and we're all apologetic and explain-y about it, the part of us that did the bad thing is no longer "out" and now a different part of us is left holding the ball, trying to explain the situation.

Yet the part of us that's now "out" doesn't *know* why we did what we did, because whatever we did was done by a different part. Our present part has no more idea about what happened than the person interrogating them!

"Why'd you do that?!" people demand of us.

"I don't know," we answer, quite genuinely.

"Yes, you do!" they insist.

But, no, "we"—"we" being the part of us they're communicating with right now—don't. We *don't* know. And the part of us that pissed everybody off is now in hiding somewhere inside us, so it's not gonna be of any help in getting us off the hook here!

This explains a lot, doesn't it?

After a late-night refrigerator raid, we wake up the next morning and ask ourselves, "Dammit, *why* the hell did I eat all that krap last night?!"

But "we" honestly don't know the answer. Because the part of us that gorged itself the night before is *not* the same part who's now moping around and punishing ourselves and trying to figure out why we could do something so counterproductive to our goals.

Except what we did the night before wasn't counterproductive to the goals of the part that did it!

Breaking News: Each of our parts have different goals! Only as we connect with them and get them into alignment with one another do their respective goals start lining up and taking us in the specific, new direction we want to go regardless of which part is "out" at any given time!

And that's exactly what we're going to discover how to do next, in Secret #8!

"You are here to enable the divine purpose of the Universe to unfold. That is how important you are!"
—Eckhart Tolle

SECRET #8:
"The Part of You That Overeats Needs a New Job"

The Job Fair

Now that you have an appreciation for the concept that we all have various parts with various talents and skills, and that these parts take turns *being us*, let's learn how to work with these parts to make our lives even more awesome!

Again, each part of us has a specific job (or group of jobs) to perform. If we have a Musical Part, it knows how to play the guitar...and piano and ukulele and any other instruments we play. Now suppose we joined a strict religion that forbade us from ever playing music again. That Musical Part would still be around, somewhere inside us, it just wouldn't get to play music any more. But—surprise, surprise—old parts (unlike dogs) *can* learn new tricks.

That very same dedication to learning and practice could be reapplied to, say, mastering a foreign language or learning to juggle. If we have a part of us that's been overeating or under-exercising or in any way actively preventing us from returning to our Ideal Body, it's time for that part to get a new job! What kind of "job"? Well, the sky's the limit! This is where we get to start thinking about all the other things we've been meaning to do all these years but were so caught up with "feeding" this one hungry part that we never quite got around to it!

396

Instead of filling up on Krap every day, our Inner Hungry-Hungry-Hippo (lulz!) will have an opportunity to undertake an entirely a new job. Best of all, this new "job" can be *anything* we desire. What would you like to do or have more of in your life on a day to day basis?

HEALTH & FITNESS
ROMANCE
WEALTH BUILDING
CREATIVITY
LEARNING A MUSICAL INSTRUMENT
EXPLORING THE WORLD
DANCING
GARDENING

Anything at all that interests you can become the new job for this already existing part of you.

Back when I was in the process of using the Parts Model to help me transition from 5 packs of cigarettes a day to 0 overnight, I referred to the inner part of me that smoked as...

Lil' Smokey
As part of my method to let go of cigarettes, I become very deliberate in deciding what job I wanted Lil' Smokey to permform for me in the future. Since I smoked so damn much, Lil' Smokey had more energy, more persistence, more drive, more daring-do and more focus than just about any other part of me.

Oh, this brings up an important point I want you to keep in mind when communicating with your *own* parts...and that is to temper your conversations with your parts with respect and appreciation and praise. I never once "confronted" Lil' Smokey and got all angry for its habit of furious chain-smoking. Quite the contrary. I let Lil' Smokey know I was in awe! How this part of me managed to find the time and the money to smoke half-a-damn-carton of cigarettes per day was almost inconceivable to me.

I repeatedly told Lil' Smokey, "Wow! You are the most incredible part of me there is! No other part of me has your endurance, your persistence, your willingness to do whatever it takes despite all sorts of obstacles. Thank you, Lil' Smokey, thank you!"

You see, my Inner Captain (and most of the other parts of me) *hated* the fact that I smoked cigarettes all the time. But Lil' Smokey was downright proud of how well he did his job!

Before I could convince Lil' Smokey to *change* jobs to something other than smoking, first I had to make sure this part of me understood that it hadn't done anything wrong and that I genuinely appreciated of all the energy it put into puffing away over the years.

Likewise, when Major Taniguchi stood in front of Lt. Onoda that fateful day on Lubang Island, surely he first commended and praised the loyal soldier for his dedication over the previous three decades, and only then did he give the Lieutenant new orders to stand down from his post.

So I spent some days just lovin' on Lil' Smokey, praising him for all his hard work of continuing to smoke cigarettes despite how unpopular and even unlawful it had become over time.

Only later did I come back and let him know that the circumstances of my life had changed and I was thinking about no longer smoking cigarettes anymore. I suggested that maybe Lil' Smokey could do something else for a change — maybe he could take on a new job.

It helped that I already had a new job in mind. I wanted to focus more and more of my energies on sharing the life-changing concepts I'd been discovering and using to help people from all walks of life heal themselves. I proposed all this to Lil' Smokey that he might pour his energies into writing, speaking and sharing the models of weight loss and personal transformation I had been developing, and he was totally down for it.

Again, our unique parts usually don't care what "game" they play — whether it's smoking or building an ultra-light glider from popsicle sticks — they just like to play.

And Lil' Smokey has been the Lil' Engine That Could for me ever since! (After all, this *is* the part that allowed "me" to write this very book you're reading of 460 pages in just 47 days from start to finish!) If anything, this part of me just seems to get stronger and stronger over time.

There's also a part of you that likes to help out others. And the way you can help me is to tell your friends and family about my book, as well as give it a sweet 5-star review on Amazon, because that will help my book rank higher (in this admittedly crowded category!) and therefore help more people fall back in love with themselves and their beautiful body!

> *"We will either find a way, or make one"*
> —Hannibal

Review of the Parts Model

We only have space to scratch the surface of how profoundly our daily actions and decisions are influenced by the various parts that make up who we are. I could easily write an entire book on the Parts Model alone — and may well do so. But for now we're primarily concerned with how our inner parts can help or hinder our goal of shedding belly fat.

The Low Carb Revolution by John McLean

Let's review how we got here...

1) Although many people think of themselves as a single, monolithic entity, in actuality we are "made up" of various parts who take turns being us

2) All humans have 7 Universal Parts that switch off performing the lion's share of all the activities we do each day (We'll do a quick overview of the 7 Universal Parts below.)

3) We each have numerous parts that are unique to us and which develop according to the circumstances of our lives. The Perfect Storm of circumstances that leads to a becoming a smoker happens for some people, and so they develop a "smoking part" and it doesn't happen for others, and so they don't.

4) If we have any kind of eating "problems" — including over-eating, binge-eating, late-night snacking, etc. — the job of doing all that chowing down is done by a part unique to us

5) Once a part joins the "team" of who we are it remains with us for life. We can starve it and ignore it for months or even years at a time, but it's always there, waiting and wanting to return.

6) If we want a part to change, we *must* give it a new "job" *(This is the most **crucial step** of all, and the one overlooked by 99.9% of conventional — or not so conventional — therapists.)*

7) Again, this new job can be anything at all, but it can't be nothing.

8) The unique part we are changing naturally *prefers* that the job be something fun and interesting. A part wouldn't be particularly excited about replacing a "negative" habit with some mindless, repetitive chore

400

like digging ditches or lawyering!

Operators Are Standing By

I'd like to invite you to begin the process of seriously thinking about what new job you'd like for the part of you that previously got "in the way" of your efforts to lose weight. Although I'm an author myself, I don't particularly recommend you *write down* a list of possible new jobs for this part.

Instead, I suggest you go for a long walk and think about potential new jobs for this part of yours. Why? Because we're trying to open up lines of communication between you and a part of you. And I can assure you straight up that your parts do not "speak" writing.

Writing is useful for communicating ideas and information to your own mind and the minds of others. Writing has no value whatsoever in communicating to your body. On the other hand, walking is something you do *with* your body. And, guess what?! The unique part of you we're trying to communicate with is also in your body, go figure!

By going for an undistracted walk (i.e., no iPod or cellphone or walking companion,, pleez!) you and your body (and along with it the part you desire to change) are now finally in the "same room" together. Is this making sense to you?

What Should I Be When I Grow Up?

So we're going to head out for a walk and come up with some ideas for a new job...or two or three!...for the formerly "over-eating" part of us to do. (Once more, "over-eating" is just shorthand for whatever way this part is preventing you from implementing the 13 progressions or otherwise holding you back from reaching the next level in your weight loss journey; it only rarely involves actual "over-eating".)

The sky's the limit—use your imagination about what kinds of new projects, behaviors and future habits you'd enjoy! Maybe you would like to…

Start a blog
Learn to salsa dance
Launch a line of natural cosmetics
Go to massage school
Volunteer more
Run for office
Run barefoot
Run away from home!

Here's a trick question for you…

Q: What's the key to successful Couples Counseling?!

A: When both members of the couple are present!

I can't tell you how many female friends I've had over the years who went to Couples Counseling to save their marriage. And when it didn't work, and they inevitably split from their partner, they would later say to me, "I think it would've been more successful if my husband had also gone." Ya think?!

Bringing Out a Part of You

So you're there, walking along, thinking about new jobs for this part. What do we want next? Obviously, we want to invite the "old" part to the dance, because the whole point of this exercise is to make actual changes within us.

How do you summon up this (or any) part?! Simply by thinking about or doing the activity its responsible for with strong intention.

If you want to summon your Inner Artist (one of the 7 Universal Parts) all you need to do is put a piece of construction paper and a box of crayons in front of your.

Believe me, your Inner Artist will be out instantaneously creating a colorful masterpiece! If you want to bring out the part of you that represents your Spirituality (another of the 7 Universal Parts), just walk into a magnificent cathedral like St. Peter's in Rome or visit one of the great wonders of the natural world, like thundering Iguacu Falls in South America, and your Spiritual side will definitely emerge, filling you with awe and humility and love!

Why do some people watch pornography?! Because doing so quickly and efficiently summons up their sexual side, which I refer to as our Inner Lover...and which is yet another of our Universal Parts.

And, for the record, I'll go ahead and list them all for you, the Universal Parts each and every one of us possess. A person might have dozens and dozens of minor parts, each of which is more or less unique to them, while we all have 7 Universal Parts that play large roles in making up Who We Are.

The 7 Universal Parts

1) Inner Lover

2) Inner Artist

3) Inner Accountant/Businessperson

4) Inner Child

5) Inner Communicator

6) Inner Healer

7) Spirituality

Okay, so backing up...you're out taking a nice stroll and your immediate goal is to summon up the part of you that "over-eats", whatever that means to you. And to do so, I want you to vividly imagine whatever action or behavior this part does for you. Again, by intensely imagining the behaviors of a part we can bring it out to play! If a smoker is trying to kick the cigarette habit on his own, by the time he starts thinking about having a cigarette, the battle is already lost...because it means: a) the part of him that smokes is now "out" and ready to do its job of smoking.

Once that side of you emerges, engage it in a conversation and let it know what's going on...how you no longer want it to do its old job but you have some ideas to propose about new jobs for it.

In other words, talk to this part of you the way you would to a friend or perhaps evern to a business partner. By the way, yes, I am literally encouraging you to talk to yourself — out loud!

Changing a Part of You

Everything we've been doing in Part Two of the *Low Carb Revolution* has fundamentally been about re-opening the lines of communication within us — whether with specific parts of us or else on a global, whole-body level.

Like Lt. Onoda, the "overeating" part of you (again, overeating is just a nominalization to describe a part that is actively working against your goal of returning to your Ideal Body) has been on a "mission" all these years, and this is your opportunity to change that mission.

You are the Captain, after all. Once you've re-established a relationship with a part and reconnected with it, the part is plenty willing to make any kind of change you desire.

So there you are, walking and talking to yourself...or, more specifically, talking to this specific part of you. Think about this part like an old friend you haven't seen in a long while. What's the first thing you wanna talk about? NOT your future plans together, but rather your past experiences...both together and separately. In other words, if this eat-a-liscious part of you were a real person you hadn't seen in forever and you ran into each other, the very first thing you'd probably talk about is stuff you did together in the past.

"Remember that time we ate that whole apple pie while the cousins were asleep?!" "Can you believe we actually downed half-a-box of Frosted Flakes without any milk?"

Catch up for a while by remembering all the good times in the past. After that, our old friend usually asks us some variation of the question, "So what have you been up to all these years?"

Now we already know what the overeating part has been up to all these years—like all parts doing their job they rarely change or alter their habit without outside influence. But WE have changed and we're continuing to change. And we need to let this part know all that because, again, like the submerged bits of an iceberg our parts don't really know what's going on in the outside world or in the rest of our lives.

So you say something along the lines of, "Hey, thanks for the great job you've done for so long of remembering to eating sugary foods all the time, but I'm now at a place in my life where I want to start losing my belly fat and ultimately return to my ideal weight. And I want your help. I want you to continue to play a big role in my life, but I want you to do something else rather than eat sugary foods for me."

And this is the point where you introduce the new job you would like this new/old chum of yours to take on.

None of this is meant to be a script to follow. I'm just giving you the *idea* of what to talk about here. If you simply keep in mind the concept that you're catching up with an old friend and then you're gonna make future plans together, then you'll be doing this exactly right!

The Next Step

With your actual friends in the real world, do you just spend time with them once every ten years or whatnot? No, you spend lots of time together, as often as possible. The closer you are, the more time you spend with one another. Some friends we can't get enough of and would hang out with every day if we could fit it into our schedule..

So too with your "new friend", the Overeating Part of you! Don't just go for a walk once and have a solitary conversation about the changes and new habits you'd like from it!

In the beginning, do this every day for a week or two. Rebuild your relationship with this part of you. The part may be a little uncertain in the beginning if you really mean it, if you genuinely want it to do completely new jobs. So it might wait until you come back again and continue to engage it in sincere dialogue about doing things differently.

Once it gets the message, one it believes you really are the Captain and this is what you really desire, only then will it make this change. So stick with it and before long you'll notice your relationship with this part of you changing right before your eyes.

This IS The Work

I shared this entire process of how to change parts with a friend of mine recently and her initial response was, "That sounds crazy!" But after a few moments she added, "But it sounds just crazy enough to be true!"

I told her, "What's the worst that can happen? You get to spend some time with yourself...and certainly everybody agrees we don't do enough of that these days!"

So I'm inviting you to give this a try. *This is the work, this is why you're here, this is why we were brought together.*

The Universe wanted you to understand how changing what you eat can change how much you weigh, and it wants you to understand that you are made up largely of various parts, many of which can be changed and transformed to create a better You. But now it's on you.

You gotta do the work. You gotta go for these walks. You gotta connect with your parts and work together to create an amazing future for the whole community of 65 trillion cells with your name attached to it!

In the very next Secret we're going to confront another insidious enemy that can sabotage our personal Revolution. This is a Trojan Horse that virtually none of the self-proclaimed "Diet Gurus" ever talk about or offer us any help with!

> *"Be kind, for everyone you meet*
> *is fighting a hard battle."*
> —Plato

SECRET #9:
"Don't Look Where You Don't Want to Go"

What Are Ya Thinking About, Baby?

There's a cardinal rule in sports like alpine skiing or bobsledding or any activity where you go downhill super fast that says, "Don't look where you don't want to go!" Because the second you start looking off to one side or another, that's exactly where you're going to end up—in the fence or over the edge! Real life is no different.

Success comes from focusing on our destination, not where we don't want to go! Maybe because we're not going quite as fast as an Olympic skier, we often don't pay much attention to where we're going. Even worse, most of us spend a lot of our time looking *only* where we don't want to go!

Here's a statistic that rocked my world when I first heard it, and I'm still feeling the after-shocks: Back in the mid-1970s, several studies discovered that up to *90% of our thoughts are negative!* Let that sink in for just a moment…

9 out of every 10 thoughts we have, all day, every day, are negative!

"I can't do that!"

"What's the point of even trying?"

"I'll never succeed at…!"

"I'm always going to be fat!"

"Who would hire me at my age?!"

"Who would date me at my age?!"

We're not talking about sometimes thinking negative thoughts about ourselves and the world around us. We're not even talking about frequently thinking negative thoughts. We're talking about the vast majority of our thoughts ending with an undesirable or unsatisfying outcome!

> *"Obstacles are those frightful*
> *things you see when you take*
> *your eyes off your goal."*
> —Henry Ford

We Are Our Own Worst Enemy

Indulge me for a moment and think about one of your best friends. Really pick somebody! Conjure up an image of her and imagine you the two are having, say, lunch together. Imagine that during lunch you relentlessly shoot down, disparage and/or disagree with almost everything she says and does.

If she expresses a deep-seated desire for a promotion at her job, you laugh and tell her not to bank on it! If she delightedly tells you she's lost 5 pounds, you feign surprise and tell her she looks more like she gained 10! If she expresses optimism about her future, you roll your eyes and loudly exclaim, "Whatever!"

Would you really treat a close friend this way? Certainly not! And if you did, you'd be looking for a new friend mighty fast!

And yet we treat *ourselves* like this—and not just during lunch, but also during breakfast and dinner and practically every moment in between! When we're relentlessly mean and negative to ourselves, what are we thinking?

I mean, seriously, what ARE we thinking?! Are we even "thinking" at all, or is something else going on? Well, we're about to find out!

"You Talking to Me?"

Here's a question for you: what is an Activity we all do pretty much every minute of the day…and yet almost never, ever, ever mention to anybody else?

No, not breathing! That's too easy! And, no, not eating—even those of us with zero self-restraint can't eat literally every minute of the day! I'll give you a hint. While you're thinking about the answer, what are you telling yourself?

Are you telling yourself, "Oh, I know, I know!" right about now? Or are you saying, "I've no idea what this bloke is prattling on about, why doesn't he just give me the bloody answer!" (Followed up quickly by saying to yourself: "And why in bleedin' hell am I suddenly talking to myself in a rubbish British accent?!")

The Answer, of course, is that each and every one of us TALKS to OURSELVES all day long…and yet we rarely even acknowledge it or ever talk about it with ourselves or with others!

As soon as we wake up in the morning the Little Voice In Our Head is already chattering away…

"Oh, great, another crummy day at my crummy job surrounded by a bunch of crummy people. I gotta find a new job. Ha! Like anybody would take a chance on me with my lack of training! I oughta exercise before work, but I'm gonna be too busy today to eat anything but Fast Food for lunch, so what's the point of even trying?" And so on and so forth.

Even the smartest, most accomplished of us of talks to himself inside his head during all the waking hours of the day like a non-stop, hyper-chatty 3 year-old!

The Little Voice in Your Head

I'm curious, have you ever once stopped and thought about the fact you talk to yourself all day long?

Have you ever confided to one of your friends, "Hey, man, I gotta tell somebody this…I got this little voice in my head, see, and it's always talking to me, see, always talking to me! The thing never shuts up, man! Am I crazy or what?!"

No, we just sorta keep the whole experience on the down low and usually never mention it to anybody. Not even to ourselves…*especially* not to ourselves!

Most feature films these days that ship on a DVD include a "Director's Commentary". If you've never experienced one, here's how they work: you watch the movie all over again with the regular soundtrack mostly muted, while the director and perhaps the writer or one of the stars talk about the process of making the actual movie — how they came up with the original idea, the adventures and misadventures of shooting it, and so on.

Even if you've never listened to a Director's Commentary, I'm sure you get the idea.

So now let's play a little game. Pretend that you bought a DVD of the blockbuster movie *Avatar*, the highest-grossing movie in history, and decide to listen to the director's commentary by James Cameron. However, instead of the typical, self-congratulatory director's commentary that you might expect, instead you were treated to a commentary track with the same 90% Negativity Factor as our personal self talk.

It might go something like this…

"Hey, Jimmy Cameron here. You'd think with all the money I've made from directing movies that I'd be happy, but I'm not. I'd tell you why I'm so unhappy,

411

but I doubt you'd care anyway. So I made this stupid movie called *Avatar* and everybody thought it was great, which just shows how dumb everybody is. I can't believe this movie made a billion dollars—I would've walked out of it myself! I wanted to cast Matt Damon instead of some unknown Australian dude and I wanted everybody to be pink but the animation company messed up and made them blue instead, etc., etc."

Wouldn't hearing Mr. Cameron trash his own movie pretty much ruin your experience of *Avatar*?! And yet we do this to ourselves all day long.

Our ongoing director's commentary of our own lives is, if anything, even more relentlessly negative than my example above.

And yet we just seem to accept "that's the way it is" and simply pretend not to notice most of the time!

The Calls Are Coming from Inside the House!

Worst of all, because our self-talk comes from INSIDE us, we tend to *believe* it unquestioningly! After all, we wouldn't lie to ourselves, would we?! (Ha, ha, ha, ha, ha!) We frequently use our internal monologue to actively discourage ourselves from trying to too hard—or to talk ourselves out of even trying at all!

Sure, trying to make any type of change in our life is scary. After all, we could fail at it.

So we hedge our bets all day long, spending a tremendous amount of our available energy just to maintain the status quo. We may not always like what we're doing right now or who we're doing it with, but at least it's *familiar* to us.

The more we can convince ourselves to keep doing exactly what we're already been doing, the more comfortable our lives will be. Or so we believe. No, the rewards won't be as great, but perhaps some of the potential risks and failures will be averted. The main problem is that we're almost completely unconscious of our pessimistic self-talk. We rarely stop to pay attention to it. We never question it or challenge it or, God forbid, talk back to it! In a moment I'll show you a simple, low-tech tool for interrupting the pattern of our negative internal monologue, but first let's broaden our canvas by going back in time.

5000 Generations Ago

Before there were words, before the first *Homo sapiens* ever created anything we would recognize as a language, we processed the world visually. Let's say you were alive 100,000 or so years ago. (My lovely children believe I actually WAS alive 100,000 years ago!)

Now pretend one fine day you're walking around, just minding your own business and thinking about remodeling the cave or something, and you suddenly see a saber-tooth tiger in the distance.

It's not close enough to be an immediate threat, but if it comes any closer you're going to need a plan of action in order to survive. Since spoken language hasn't been invented yet, you have no Little Voice in your Head to tell you what to do. Instead, your brain does one of its favorite tasks, it "remembers" by playing a series of visual images from your past...sorta like movie trailers, except projected inside your head.

In this case, your brain remembers seeing an animal like this before. A saber-tooth tiger recently ate your best friend Grok while he was lifting barbell-shaped rocks and you now "learn" from that experience by playing a short movie in your head.

Then your brain replays the scenario again, only this time you are the one being eaten rather than poor ol' Grok!

Next your brain quickly imagines several possible futures, one right after the other: In the first imagined future, you fight the saber-tooth tiger with your new & improved Rock, ver. 2.0 and win! In the second imagined future, the Rock just bounces off the saber-tooth tiger and you endure the same fate as hapless Grok! In the third imagined future, you run away and live to fight another day! And in the fourth imagined future, Grok's widow sees you running away, decides you're a coward and declines to take you for a mate!

Based on your own particular strengths and experience, you *believe* one of these internal movies more than the others and base your actions in the real world accordingly.

In this case, you RUN! And Grok's widow does not see you run away and the two of your settle down and live happily ever after! (I mean, why not?!)

To this very day we still process the world fundamentally like our hunter-gatherer ancestors — running movies in our head all day long *rehearsing* potential successes or failures in every situation we face. Then and now, the human mind ceaselessly creates still images and/or movies in an ongoing attempt to understand the world and predict the outcome of our current activity.

And just as with our internal monologue, we use these "rehearsal movies" to imagine ourselves *failing* far more often than we imagine ourselves succeeding. Once again, we fail in our mental movies approximately 90% of the time!

> *"Anxiety is nothing...but repeatedly*
> *imagining failure in advance"*
> —Seth Godin

Coming Soon to a Brain Near You

When your average person pictures themselves on a first date or at a job interview or standing in front of the Pearly Gates, their internal movies and monologue more often than not feature them being turned down, rejected and even condemned to the other place!

What does that mean for anyone who has ever struggled to lose weight? It means that while most overweight people *say* they are sick of being overweight and want to return to their Ideal Body, that's just what they are saying on the outside, to other people.

On the inside, it's a different story, isn't it?! Deep within us our negative internal movies and dialogue paint a gloomy picture of deprivation, guilt and probable failure.

> *"Our imagination is like the*
> *previews for the coming*
> *attractions of our life"*
> — Albert Einstein

Righting The Ship

When you're fighting a revolution, there cannot be any room for doubt about the outcome. We've drawn a line in the sand. We've announced to the world that our body is worth fighting for.

Now we need to do something about our unhelpful and counter-productive internal movies and monologue. We're going to do this in steps, in a series of progressions—because, as we well know, that's the way we learn every complicated thing we ever learn!

Our first progression in this task is to get a handle on one very specific type of inner movie and self-talk. And that means the negativity we heap upon ourselves

415

about our bodies and our (in)ability to return to our natural state of our Ideal Body.

When the ship's taking on water, the best first step is to learn how to bail! Only then can we begin righting the ship and sailing in a bold new direction in our life! I'm about to share with you a technique for expanding your awareness of what's going on inside your own head and enable you to make dramatic changes in your results, simply by getting out of your own way! And it all starts with a *rubber-band!*

At this juncture when I'm working with private clients I hand them a big, colorful bag of rubber-bands and ask them to pick a color they like and a size that fits comfortably around their wrist.

Perhaps you've got a rubber band laying around somewhere — in your desk drawer at work or wrapped around last week's unread newspaper or holding the broccoli stems together in your fridge. If so, grab one of them little suckers and put it around your wrist so you can play along at home!

The Rubber-Band Technique

The Rubber-Band Technique that I'm about to share with you is simplicity itself! We're going to use a rubber-band to monitor the things we tell ourselves and the pictures/movies we screen in our minds regarding only a single aspect of our lives — implementing the 13 Progressions of the *Low Carb Revolution* and returning to our Ideal Body!

One of the big reasons that so many fine people never actually lose any weight is they talk themselves out of it before they even start!

"There's no point in even trying anymore"

"Just one waffle won't hurt"

"It's gonna be too hard"

"I can't do this because I'm too stressed out right now"

"I can always lose weight next year"

What I teach my private clients to do is to start by deliberately paying attention to their self-talk and their internal movies *only* regarding their imagined success or failure at losing weight.

If they notice themselves saying or imagining to themselves any negative outcome or failure regarding their transition back to their birthright of living at their Ideal Body, they are to simply SNAP the rubber-band to interrupt their pattern, and then deliberately tell themselves or visualize a positive, successful outcome...

"This is easier than I imagined!"

"Nothing tastes as good as thin feels!"

"I enjoy living in a leaner, healthier body!"

"I feel safe and loved as I continue to lose weight!"

What could be easier than that?! Just notice your thoughts regarding eating and your weight. If your internal monologue/movies are positive, keep up the good work! If they're negative, SNAP the rubber band to interrupt your pattern

Then immediately and deliberately fashion an opposite (that is to say, positive) statement/movie to communicate to yourself.

Remember, at the start we're concerned only with your internal monologue and movies related to reaching your Ideal Body.

As I tell my smoking-cessation clients, "For the first two weeks focus only on curbing your self-sabotaging thoughts about letting go of cigarettes. Feel completely free to continue telling yourself that you're lazy or unproductive or prudish or any other unwarranted self-criticism you desire! Or...NOT!"

Once you get a "handle" on your thoughts/movies regarding this one aspect of your life that you want to change, then you can pick the next area of your life to work on and before you know it you'll become part of a frighteningly small minority of folks who talk to themselves mostly in loving, supporting and accepting terms.

A Head Start!

Lest the idea of monitoring your negative self-talk on even the single topic of finally losing those excess pounds still seem daunting to you, here's a final reminder that I've created a valuable tool for you that will do a lot of the heavy-lifting for you.

Visit the link below to gain immediate access to the FREE bonus *Low Carb Affirmations,* an mp3 audio module designed to support your journey. Containing powerful, positive statements about loving yourself, loving your body and letting go of your excess weight, these affirmations effectively help drown out your negative inner monologue while you're listening to them.

That's why I strongly encourage you to take advantage of this unique tool and listen to the recording as often as possible.

Of course, I'm using the word "listen" loosely, since you never have to sit down and focus your attention on them the way you would with, say, an Audiobook. Instead, just play them in the background, the way some people leave the radio or TV playing in the other room all day long.

And the affirmations can be played at a volume that's so low it won't be distracting. Even if you can barely, hardly hear them, these powerful, positive statements about your ability to succeed at losing weight this time around and create the healthy lifestyle you desire and deserve will penetrate deep down inside you and help you transform yourself from the inside out.

Best of all, the *Low Carb Affirmations* I created for you contain a Dual-Hemisphere pattern. This consists of two separate, overlapping audio tracks—one for each hemisphere of your brain. Listening to these affirmations is a key to your success and I strongly recommend you take advantage of them whenever you can. Believe me, all sorts of goodness will flow from listening to them as often as possible!

http://db.tt/69WOj7pW

Coming up in Secret #10...we're going to start asking some important questions about what's next for you. Because returning to your Ideal Body isn't the end of your journey, it's really just the beginning. So we're gonna start planning ahead for the next chapter in your wonderful life!

"It's not your job to like me, it's mine"
—Byron Katie

SECRET #10:
"You're Either IN The Revolution... or You're WATCHING It!"

Your Life is Not A Dress Rehearsal

During the never-ending nightmare of my decades-long imprisonment in my own personal Smoke-catraz, I kept telling myself, "I'll quit next week!" or "I'll quit right before the reunion!" or "I'll quit once I get out of this relationship...or once I get into a relationship...or instead of being in a relationship!"

Because my thinking was so clouded by cigarette smoke, for years and years I had the mind-set that my Life hadn't really started yet, that this time "didn't count", that I'd get things going pretty soon now! Pretty, pretty, pretty soon, as Larry David is wont to say in the HBO series *Curb Your Enthusiasm*! And so the years passed.

Those of us trapped in the chronic embrace of cigarettes or carbohydrates tend to lie. We lie to others...and we lie to ourselves.

One day during my Mad Scientist phase I had an epiphany: most of the stuff I told myself was an outright falsehood.

My self-communication consisted primarily of one lie after another from morning til night. So I decided not to lie to myself for the next 24 hours. And I probably learned more about myself during those 24 hours than during all the previous years of my life!

One of my most life-changing realizations was that

I'd allowed myself to become *content* with just sitting in the audience. Yet...being content is no way to go through life! The biggest obstacle to enjoying a spectacular life is to have a decent life, right?!

Young people often think Hate is the opposite of Love. Whereas anybody who's been married before will tell you differently. The opposite of Love is more often...Apathy. Because Apathy leads us to become content to stay in a relationship, or content to leave it, content to gain weight or content to lose it. We just don't give a damn one way or the other anymore.

> *"My great concern is not whether*
> *you failed, but whether you are*
> *content with your failure"*
> — Abraham Lincoln

Life is Not a Spectator Sport

The moment I grokked that I had been *content* doing what I was doing with my life — which was, honestly, pretty much nothing up until that point — was the moment I finally started to wake up!

Now in my defense, when you're smoking upwards of 5 packs of cigarettes per day and your diet consists of about 110% carbohydrates, there's not much else you CAN do other than sit around during recess and watch all the other kids play! Yet I did gain enough clarity during that one day of only telling myself the Truth (what a novel concept!) that I realize I had two fundamental options in my life...

OPTION I

I could continue to hide from myself and the world in my self-imposed prison of carbohydrates and cigarette smoke...while living primarily in my head.

or

OPTION II

I could find some way to get out of my head and back into my body so I could join the Revolution — or maybe even start my own one day!

> *"Every single successful person I've ever spoken to has a Turning Point. The turning point was when they made a clear, specific, unequivocal decision they were not going to live like this anymore; they were going to achieve success. Some people make that decision at 15 and some make it at 50, but most people never make it at all"*
> — Brian Tracy

The End is Just the Beginning

Now is the time for you to start planning for the life you really desire after you've reached your goal and lost your excess belly fat.

You've known all along that returning to your Ideal Body wouldn't be the end of the story, but merely the beginning!

After all, if you and your partner are pregnant, when you eventually go to the hospital to deliver the baby, you don't leave the baby there and return home, saying, "Okay, well that's over with!"

No, bringing baby home is just the beginning of the Party! All the fun is yet to come! (Until they become teenagers…but that's a whole different story!)

You Don't Need No Stinkin' Goals!

What, no goals?! Yes, yes, yes, I know that *everybody* and their aunt says you're supposed to *write down your goals!*

Apparently "they" polled every human who ever lived, and the ones who wrote down their goals all became multi-millionaires, philanthropists and jet-setters by the age of thirty. Meanwhile, the ones who didn't write down their goals became overweight, unproductive crack-head bums living on the street.

Or at least that's what everybody (and their aforementioned aunt) would have you believe. And they may even be right. Despite all that, I absolutely, positively, 100% do NOT recommend that you write down your goals.

Your mind loves lists—but not for the reason you might think. Lists don't help remind the brain to do something in the future, they *train your brain to forget!* Making a list is a super convenient way to store information *outside* of yourself. A list is nothing more than a low-tech flash drive—one of those cheap, almost disposal memory storage devices you plug right into the side of your computer.

As soon as you "transfer" information to a list, then your brain doesn't have to bother thinking about it any more. It simply needs to remember where you put the piece of paper with the info written on it. If you write down a phone number or the winning lottery numbers that appeared to you in a dream, you don't ever have to bother learning or remembering that information anymore.

Writing down your goals means generating a list of stuff you wanna do with your life that exists outside of you, where you don't have to remember it and so it has no real chance of having any particular impact on your behaviors and actions.

Don't get me wrong, making lists can be highly valuable! If you're headed to the grocery store, by all means make a list. And if you are Santa Claus,, make a list and even check the damn thing twice! But while writing down a list is a lovely way to supplement our ridiculously limited short-term memory, it's not at all a useful tool for generating the enthusiasm and passion that our mind, body and spirit require to create an entirely new reality for ourselves. The best way to influence ourselves while creating emotion is through listening to and telling Stories!

We Are Story-Telling Machines

I lived in Dallas in my early twenties after graduating from college. I was quite the film buff in those days, and one day I decided to write a screenplay for a feature-length film. The story involved the comic adventures of a temporary secretary — which was seemingly the only job for which my degree in Literature & Languages from the University of Texas had qualified me!

I'd written maybe half of the script when one day I suddenly stopped in my tracks. I realized that I was writing down all these words for *actors* to say, yet I had almost zero acting experience in my own life apart from inconsequential roles in a couple of high school plays.

At that moment, I decided to go out and do some acting, reasoning (correctly, as it turned out) that acting would make me a better screenplay writer.

I also decided my acting needed to be on stage. My belief — then and now — was that "real" actors work in theatre, while "pretend" actors do movies and "non" actors appear in commercials. In those pre-Internet days, I read (in an actual newspaper, mind you!) about an audition for a stage version of Ken Kessey's wonderful, surreal novel, *One Flew Over The Cuckoo's Nest* and decided to go try out.

There was only one problem: I didn't know the first thing about acting or how to audition or anything of that nature!

The Low Carb Revolution by John McLean

*"If at first you don't succeed, think how may
people you've made happy!"*
—H. Duane Black

Fake It 'til You Make It

A year or so earlier, during my senior year at UT, I scored one of the more enviable living situations of any male college student in the United States. I was the sole male roommate in a spacious, semi-haunted house along with 4 beautiful, female University of Texas Drama students. (What a krazy life I've led, now that I think back on it!)

Even though I wasn't an actor back then, nor had I ever taken a single acting class, I *did* get to spend an entire year around my actor roommates and their legions of gay and straight theatre friends. (I'm just kidding about them having any *straight* theatre friends!)

So before heading over to the *One Flew Over The Cuckoo's Nest* audition that day, I decided that even though I wasn't myself an actor, if I simply *acted* like the actors I knew then maybe the casting people would be fooled into thinking I, too, was an actual actor.

But then I realized I had another little problem I was aware that actual actors presented themselves at auditions with their acting resume typed out on a piece of paper which was stapled to the back of a headshot. The headshot itself was supposed to be a glossy, 8" x 10" photograph, usually taken by professional photographers who make quite a handsome living by preying on this one little desperate subset of humanity!

Sooth to say, I didn't have a professional headshot. In fact, other than stacks of Polaroids of my Dad and I during our many travels around Europe and Asia, I had no photographs of myself at all. So I improvised!

In lieu of a standard B&W photograph, I simply took a piece of 8x10 inch cardstock and, using a bright blue Sharpie, I drew a narrow oval for my head, added dots for my eyes and nose, a curve for my mouth, and then a bunch of little circles for my then long, flowing curly hair. With my own unique "headshot" in hand, I drove to the audition. Once there, I simply pretended like I knew what I was doing.

And it worked! It actually worked! They cast me in their play!

Now I played an exceedingly minor character in the show, a nutcase named Scanlon, and I only had a single line—a line I anxiously anticipated and rehearsed saying about four thousand times each night before actually uttering it during the show! But...as one of the "loonies" I was on stage virtually the entire show and I lost any fear of being on stage...AND I started learning how to act just by paying attention during the weeks of rehearsals...AND I got to hang around experienced actors for the entire show, which was the best training of all.

Footnote: It's customary in the theatre world to display the headshots of the thespians involved in the play on a wall in the lobby or such. During the run of *One Flew Over The Cuckoo's Nest* my hand-drawn with blue Sharpie "headshot" got more attention than all of the other actors' professional headshots combined!

All's Well That Ends Well

That was my first acting experience, but far from my last. Over the years I went on to act in dozens of plays, often in starring roles—the highlight being one of the lead roles in Charles Busch's outrageous comedy, *Vampire Lesbians of Sodom.*

In addition, I studied with a number of well-known teachers in Dallas, Los Angeles and Austin. And later still, I wrote, directed and acted in two independent, comic feature films shot in and around Austin. And all of this acting and creativity started with a story.

Three stories, actually. First, the story I was originally writing in the form of a script about a temporary secretary. Second, a story I told myself about how going out and learning to act might have the secondary benefit of making me a better screenwriter. And third, a story about faking it 'til you make it—which is as true as it is cliché!

Humans are indeed story-telling machines. I could easily write an entire book about "Acting For Beginners" and fill it with the treasure trove of auditioning and acting techniques (which are actually two completely different disciplines, I hasten to add) that I've learned over the years.

But, honestly, pretty much every "lesson" you need to learn in order to go out and audition for your very first play are included in the story I just told you about my debut theatrical experience.

By the way, I can sum up everything you need to know about *acting* in a single phrase…a phrase that seems laughably simple and easy to achieve, but which in reality requires years of study and practice to pull off.

Wanna learn the Secret to Acting in one phrase? Well, here 'tis…

Stand still, don't act.

Stories Have "Legs"

Lists come and go, but *stories* remain with us. How many times have you seen your friends express concern and even genuine sadness whenever a real, live natural disaster strikes the world?

For the most part, however, they're not usually sad to the point of crying about it unless the disaster struck very close to home, are they?!

But then these same friends go to a movie about a

pretend disaster that never actually happened in the real world and cry like little babies when an actor they like pretends to die in the pretend disaster!

Completely made-up stores impact our central nervous system just as powerfully—and sometimes more so—than that little thing called reality! Instead of a writing down an easy-to-forget "list" of our goals, instead we're going to do something that's much simpler and far more effective in shaping our possible future.

We're going to tell a story! A story about ourselves and our life as we successfully let go of our belly fat, return to our Ideal Body and begin waking up to our full potential in the world!

The Vision Letter

When I stumbled upon this little exercise it changed virtually everything I believed about what my future might hold in store for me...and I humbly submit that your results may be every bit as earth-shattering! This process is called writing a "Vision Letter", which is simply a letter to someone other than yourself, describing your life.

The catch is that you write it from the *Future*. Of course, you won't actually GO into the Future (though if you've discovered the technology to do that, please tell the Future we all said, "Hi"!) Instead, you're going to do what your brain likes doing most: *pretend*!

Here's how it works. To create your Vision Letter, simply...

1) Set aside a quiet time with pen and paper

2) Address the letter to a real or imaginary friend

3) Magically transport yourself in your mind a year or a decade into your future

4) Write down in the letter whatever you imagine your life is like in the future

5) Return to the present and contemplate what you've written

And that's all there is to it! Imagine your life at some point in the future and write it down. You don't have to spend a lot of time doing this—writing a one or two page letter is plenty to get the flavor of it hot.

When I wrote my first vision letter, I sat down at my desk and took out pen and paper. (By the way, to get the maximum impact from this experience, please write this letter by hand, the old-fashioned way, and not on any kind of electronic device!) At the top of the first page I wrote…

"Dear Hanna…"

Now Hanna is one of my very best friends and she was the lead actor in my second feature film—a crazy, feature-length musical comedy called *Z: A Zombie Musical*. Hanna is beautiful, brilliant and uninhibited. I don't know why I picked Hanna over anybody else to write my Vision Letter to, other than the fact that she's the sort of person who will always love me no matter what.

Then I just started writing, describing my life in the "present". And by present I mean the future. I mentally transported myself into my future—I think it was about five years ahead.

Without ever once stopping to think about or judge with my conscious mind what I was doing, I simply wrote down various aspects of my life as I imagined them. I described to Hanna the city I lived in. (To my surprise, it was a city I'd never really thought about moving to!) I described my house and my relationships. I described new healing techniques I'd created, books I had written and online products I had created. After a page and a half—perhaps fifteen or twenty minutes of writing, in total—I stopped. I was done. And I was, frankly, amazed.

The future I'd described for myself was so attractive, so alluring and so perfect for me. I realized instantly that it was exactly the future I desired...and exactly the future I intended to create for myself. By crafting it as a letter, it seemed more like a story in my mind, a story I was telling an intimate friend.

Because stories have something no list can ever possess: *emotion*!

And unlike writing down a list of goals (which I would've had to refer back to again and again to remember what to do) just by imagining and writing down my Vision Letter, it immediately became a permanent part of me.

Remember how I used a blue Sharpie to draw a stick figure headshot of myself for my first acting audition?! Of course you do! Because you learned about it in the context of a *story*, and so you're likely to remember that little detail for a good, long time!

I never actually went back to re-read that Vision Letter since that day, because I didn't have to! The story I told in my letter was so engraved in my mind that it continues to live on there quite nicely without any additional reminders! I like to think you will have a similarly constructive experience when you create your own Vision Letter.

What's YOUR Story?

Okay, we've got another homework assignment here. As you've surely divined, the task at hand is to write your own Vision Letter.

If you're genuinely serious about one day changing your story and making the transition back to your

430

natural state of your Ideal Body, then creating a Vision Letter and having a sense of your beautiful, healthy *future* is imperative. I'd like for you to set aside some time in the very near future (like, for example, today!) to do this simple exercise.

Address the letter to someone who cares about you or even an imaginary person or someone from a movie or book. Then use your imagination to time-travel a few years ahead and let your "friend" know what's going on in your new, improved, lemon-scented life of the future. And for goodness sakes, remember to mention right up front about your success in letting go of your belly fat and achieving all your weight loss goals!

You might even start your letter by saying, "It's now been x years since we last saw each other…and you won't believe how much weight I've lost and how amazing I look and feel these days!" Then just go from there!

You Gotta Do the Work!

Don't simply *tell yourself* you're gonna do this later—I want you to *commit* to it! I want you to promise you'll play this game.

In fact, I want you to promise OUT LOUD! It's been known since ancient times that saying things out loud somehow helps bring them to life in the world in a way far more profound than when they're still mere thoughts inside our noggins.

Please read the following sentence out loud…

"I promise to create the time and space for myself sometime within the next 24 hours to write a Vision Letter about my beautiful, exciting future!"

Did you read it out loud? That wasn't so difficult, was it? *Committing* to do the work is often harder than actually doing the work! Now that you've made a commitment, the hardest part is over!

In the next Secret we're going to discover one of the foundational principles of the revolutionary change-work I've developed...the significance of getting out of our heads and into our bodies!

> *"Nothing great was ever accomplished*
> *without enthusiasm!"*
> —Mary Kay Ash

SECRET #11:
"Get Out of Your Head...and Into Your Body"

The Party is in Your Body!

Modern humans have become obsessed with their minds to a degree that's not, well, normal. The truth is...most of us live in our heads most of the time. We THINK too much. Not only do we think too much, but we often even *think* about thinking too much!

One of the leading reasons that upwards of 70% of Americans are, shall we say, *over-nourished* is because we've become completely disconnected from our bodies and have retreated into our heads. I mean, how do most of us spend our free time? Watching television, playing on the internet, reading magazines, texting one another, etc. All of which are activities done by and for the mind. Our brains have become addicted to being informed and/or entertained during all the waking hours of our day. We get "bored" in about *pi* seconds if our poor conscious mind isn't distracted by some form of entertainment or another. We resent waiting even half a minute for the elevators doors to open because they offer nothing to occupy our attention!

On top of that, many of us devote considerable amounts of thought to the negative or positive changes we'd like to make in our life: lose weight, learn how to play the double-belled euphonium, etc. The problem with that, of course, is that *thought* is what our mind does. Losing weight, playing the double-belled euphonium and any other amazing outcomes we desire in our life are usually the realm of the body!

And yet for most of us our bodies are, at best, merely an afterthought in our lives.

We've been exploring a radical new theory of habits in this book based on an understanding that our habits are run by our body, and not by our mind the way we've always been taught.

Transforming our habits—whether eliminating negative ones or adopting positive ones—requires us to involve and engage our body in the process.

Because... the Party Is In Your Body!

As you learn to appreciate and love your beautiful body once again, you'll find that it can seem downright easy to lose any and all the excess weight you desire. I want to share with you a story.

At first this might seem like a story about monkeys, but don't be fooled. This is not a story about monkeys. *This is a story about your body!*

> *"Great ideas originate in the muscles"*
> —Thomas Edison

The Four Monkeys

Once upon a time a group of researchers created an unusual experiment. They took four monkeys and put them in a sealed room with glass walls so they could be observed. In the middle of the room was a pole with a sort of shelf on the very top of it.

From time to time, a delightful snack would be placed by a robotic arm on the shelf at the top of the pole—and one or several of the monkeys would scramble up it to get the scrumptious treat. The monkeys quickly developed the habit of climbing the pole whenever they heard the tell-tale whir of the robotic arm setting the extra food into place.

Then one day the researchers changed things up, as researchers are wont to do. Exactly at the same time as the usual feast arrived on the pole's shelf and the monkeys clambered towards it, several water jets spraying pressurized, ice-cold water began firing at the top of the pole, repelling the monkeys away from the snack and leaving them drenched and shivering.

Confused, the monkeys tried a few more times to reach the snacks, but in each case they were blasted off the pole by the cold, pressurized water stream. Finally the dazed monkeys gave up trying to reach the snack altogether and retreated to a corner of the room. Somewhat later, another portion of the special food was placed atop of the pole. One of the bolder monkeys made a game effort at climbing up to it—but again the ice-cold water blasted his furry butt right off the pole and he failed as well.

After just a few sessions of this, the monkeys had learned their lesson.

They developed a brand new habit...whenever treats appeared atop the pole, they screeched and ducked into a corner of the room, as far away as they could from the possibility of being blasted by freezing water, and then just sat there, staring forlornly at the unreachable food at the top of the pole.

Okay, so monkeys can learn habits, like climbing a pole to get food, and they can also learn new habits, like not climbing the pole despite the presence of food.

There's a name for this latter habit. It's called "Learned Helplessness". We've all been there—but that's still not the point of our story yet!

In fact, here's where it starts to really get interesting.

The New Monkey

One day, one of the four monkeys was removed from the room. In his place a new monkey was added — a monkey that none of the other three had ever seen before. Not long after the new monkey's arrival, the old drill began again.

Food appeared at the top of the pole and the new monkey began to climb towards it. However he didn't make it very far...the three original monkeys physically grabbed the new fella and hauled him back down, shrieking and pointing and somehow communicating in Monkey-ease that under no circumstances was the new monkey to try to climb the pole for the food. As long as no monkey reached the top of the pole, the icy water jets didn't fire and everybody stayed dry — albeit a bit hungrier. After just a couple of repetitions of being pulled off the pole by the others, the new monkey also learned a new habit: stay away from the treats on the pole.

So far, so good, but now it gets even better. One by one, each of the original monkeys was taken out of the room and replaced by a new monkey.

Eventually, all the monkeys in the room were new monkeys. Treats continued to regularly appear atop the pole, but the "new" monkeys avoided it so they won't be punished with the ice-cold blast of — hey wait a second!

None of these are the original monkeys!

That means *none* of these monkeys EVER had the actual experience of being blasted by the high-pressure, ice-cold water.

None of these monkeys has any memory or direct knowledge of *why* they aren't allowed to climb the pole and get the treats in the first place.

Yet they still don't climb the pole and they don't get

the treats.

The researchers even turned off the water cannons completely so there wouldn't be any repercussions if the monkeys suddenly decided to go after the food, but the monkeys continued to stick to their habit of "Learned Helplessness" and never again attempted to claim the food at the top of the pole.

How many of *us* do something very similar? How many times have we been held back from trying something new or coloring outside the lines because of dire warnings and discouragements from the other little "monkeys" in our Tribe?!

How many of us act just like the monkeys and do the exact same things to *ourselves*? Especially in our bodies. Well, to be more specific, to our cells!

We're about to go for one final swim in the ocean of science-osity, but it's all for a good cause (hint: YOU), so stick with me, baby!

> *"We don't see things as they are,*
> *we see things as we are"*
> — Anaïs Nin

What Are Cells?

Cells are actually pretty cool. All life is made from cells. Period. If it's alive, it's got at least one cell, and usually more. Cells are the smallest units of life on Earth, and can do everything any plant or animal can do, only at a more primitive level, naturally.

If you take a cell from any plant or animal in the world—or, for that matter, take any single cell from your own body—and put it in the vicinity of a nutrient, the cell will find a way to propel itself close enough to ingest the food source. Similarly, if you put that single cell near a toxin, the cell will attempt to move away.

Any individual cell from your body has a primitive

circulatory system and skeleton. It can digest nutrients and excrete waste. (Everything poops...even cells!) A lone cell also has the functional equivalent of a nervous system and immune system and it can even reproduce itself.

Single cells are just like me and you, only lots smaller! They're sort of like our own personal Mini-Me's!

And, most importantly, a cell has the ability to *learn* from its micro-environment (that is to say, what's going on immediately around it) and change its behaviors and actions accordingly. In other words, just like monkeys and people, cells can *learn* to abandon old habits and adopt new ones.

> *"Like humans, single cells analyze thousands*
> *of stimuli from their environment...and are*
> *capable of learning from their experiences and*
> *creating cellular memories, which they pass*
> *on to their offspring."*
> —Bruce Lipton, Ph.D.

The Cambrian Explosion

For the first 4 billion or so years of our planet's existence, all life consisted of single-cell organisms.

ALL life!

Nothing was more than one cell each! For 4 BILLION years!

For the vast, vast majority of time since the creation of our planet some 4.7 billion years ago, single cells *were* life!

Then one day the most amazing thing happened. Perhaps it was a sunny Thursday in April. Maybe around tea time. Whenever it was, and for whatever reason, two of these basic units of life called cells suddenly decided to "hang out" together on a more or less permanent basis.

They somehow learned that if they got together and shared the workload of finding food, avoiding danger, excreting waste, reproducing and the like, then their chances of survival would dramatically increase. At that moment, "merely" 600 million years ago, the first multi-cellular organism on Earth was born.

Now as a survival strategy, pairing up two separate cells proved to be best idea ever. (Granted, this was the first new idea in over 4 billion years, so there wasn't much competition back then!)

Before long, all the cool kids in the ocean—and the ocean, by the way, is where literally everybody lived— were hooking up in twos...then threes...and before you know it there were new life forms made up of hundreds and then thousands of cells.

Having bunches of other cells to share the workload with also meant that some of the cells could specialize. There could be cells that formed a primitive stomach that could hold lots of food at once...so this new multi-cellular organism no longer had to eat constantly, but could now spend time doing other stuff. Other cells might specialize to become fins to move around more efficiently in the dense seas. And there could be cells that acted like a poison to ward off other, larger groups of cells that might come along to eat you. Little by little, new, improved and amazingly diverse life forms appeared...all of them made out of bunches (and bunches!) of cells.

Within a mere 50 million years—a blink of the eye in geological terms—the forefathers and foremothers of virtually *all* plant and animal life we know today was born.

Flowers, fauna and fungi, sharks and whales, mammals and birds, all of these and more got their start during this unprecedented era of cellular creativity.

Termed the "Cambrian Explosion", in this ridiculously short span of time, cells learned that building highly complex communities with like-minded cells was the only way to fly!

Now let's fast-forward 600 million years until we arrive back at the present day and let's talk about *you*. Because, after all, YOU are the Hero of this entire story...and have been all along! But if we are to talk about you, that leads us to another question.

Who Are "You"?

Take a moment, if you please, and look down at your left hand. (Really do this. Please!) Now trace your eyes along the length of your arm and across your body and down your right leg and notice your right foot, or at least the shoe/flip-flop/glass slipper containing your right foot! You're all of a piece, aren't you? Cut from whole cloth, as the lofty poets might say.

If you are like most people, you've gone through life thinking of your physical body as a single, monolithic entity known as "you"—a perfect example of one entire, whole and complete Human Being, right? Ummmm, not so fast!

We are a complex community of parts, both on the inside and on the outside. We've already discovered that we're all made of parts who take turns being us: astronaut, lover, father, dancer, serial killer, etc.

But it's also true that our physical bodies are made up of parts...lots and lots of them! If you were to scratch the surface of your body, you would find that you're no different than any other plant or animal on the globe—which is to say you are thriving, bustling *community* of single cells which have thrown in their lot together.

In fact, it takes about 60 TRILLION individual cells

to make up one You!

Each and every one of the trillions of cells in your body is fully capable of surviving on its own, but it is more likely to survive a good bit longer and have a better quality of life if it remains with the rest of the class.

After all, any single cell from you can find nourishment, avoid danger, poop etc., but it's not liable to ever figure out a way to get on a plane and travel to a sexy Caribbean island for a well-deserved vacation!

Who's The Boss?

So you're made up of trillions upon trillions of cells, but who's in charge of all of them. Who's the boss?! Why, *you're* the boss! You are the Emperor of the community of cells that bears your name. You are the Captain, the Master, the Chief, the Leader, the Ruler, the Potentate, the Grand high Poo-Bah of a total population of 60-odd trillion inhabitants. Welcome to "YOU"!

And "you" consist of an amazing community of these trillions of cells, each of them working in harmony-ish to create the experience of "you" in this world! In the next Secret, you'll learn how virtually every single one of the 60 trillion cells that go into making one of You gets replaced on a regular schedule. Some of your cells live only a few days before being replaced…while others live for a bit longer.

But sooner or later, pretty much all of them get replaced. In fact, most of the cells in your *current* body have been replaced many, many, many times over! Physically, you are no longer the same person you were when you were born.

Virtually every cell that made up "you" when you were just a wee lad or lass are long gone and others have taken their place…and others have taken their place, and so on! In fact, as we'll discover soon enough,

441

you're not even physically the same person now you were at this time last year!

> *"Knowledge is only a rumor until you get it*
> *in your muscles"*
> —Robert Dilts

Cellular Learnings

Each of our trillions of cells can learn how to change their behaviors and functions to respond to what's going on around them. The cells that make up who we are learn stuff all the time. Some of the stuff they learn helps us and some of it doesn't.

Now just as you may know your hometown like the back of your hand, but have no clue what the people and culture are like in, say, the Icelandic capital of Reykjavik, so too the cells lining your stomach aren't exactly keeping up with the latest haps of the specialized cells in your right ear drum.

If you're on Facebook you may have 500 or even 5000 friends, let's say...but in truth you can really keep tabs on only about *150* or so of them. (By the way, this theoretical upper limit of 150-ish friends whom we can realistically remain in close, personal contact with is known as "Dunbar's Number", and is a well-documented, cross-cultural phenomena among humans!)

So you or I can only ever really know about 150 people, yet there are now over 850 MILLION Facebook users!

We are all part of the same online social networking community known as Facebook, but the vast majority of us will never have a relationship with the vast majority of the other Facebook users. Keeping up with the approximately 150 members in our own Tribe is about all that we have bandwidth for.

And the exact same principle applies to your busy cells. They're good pals with lots of other cells in their immediate micro-environment, but they don't personally know all 60 trillion cells in your entire body. The complete lack of communication between most of the cells in your body helps explain why old-fashioned diets are often such spectacular failures.

What happens when we hear about some new fad diet?! Our brains learn all the nuances of it, but none of the cells in our body are even aware of what we're doing. Nobody ever told *them* about the diet!

After getting little or no results after a week or a month on our new regime, we toss it in the garbage pail and go back to our originally scheduled programming of carbs, starches and food-shaped chemicals. That's how many of us become overweight! We get in the habit of eating a certain way and still erroneously believe that we can change our habits by changing our mind!

The Buck Stops at Our Cells

As we've explored in some detail here in the *Low Carb Revolution*, our habits are controlled by our body. And we now know that our body isn't one big, monolithic super-entity, but is a community of trillions, which is organized just like we organize ourselves on this planet.

Most of us live in neighborhoods and those neighborhoods are located along with a bunch of other ones in a particular city, which is in a certain province or state that contains other cities, which is in a particular country that has lots of provinces or states and so on.

When habits are learned by your body, it's not your whole body that learns the habit, but rather some of the "cell citizens" in a very specific little neighborhood. If you ever smoked cigarettes, then you might recall that whenever it was Time to have a smoke, you usually experienced a sort of craving sensation or pang, perhaps somewhere in your chest or stomach area...or maybe on your tongue or in your jaw.

These "pangs" were caused by a small collection of cells in some particular neighborhood sending you a specific message: light one up. Now, when you first decided to quit, your mind might have known you were quitting...but until the actual cells responsible for the "pang" receive and accept the message that you want to quit smoking they'll continue to produce the physical sensations urging you to indulge your habit.

Similarly, the actual cells in our tummy that send us a signal urging us to pull into the McTacoHut drive thru for some hot, steaming Krap fresh from the Fry-o-later where they haven't changed the oil since the Eisenhower administration are merely firing because of their current orders. Our stomach cells don't know that Krap creates health problems and weight gain and that our Fat Food lifestyle is killing us, they're just doing what they learned to do from the cells who came before them—no less than the new monkeys in the room learned the habit of not climbing the pole without ever learning why.

Is this making sense? The reason we often stay overweight is because once any one of our cells learns a new strategy or habit, it tends to keep on doing it.

That particular cell doesn't know whether or not its behavior serves the greater good of the whole community of cells (i.e., you) because it's not exactly on speaking terms with the other 59, 999,999,999 cells!

However, there IS someone who *can* be on speaking terms with every single cell.

You Are The Grand Poo-Bah

You are ultimately in charge of your body. By your "Body" I mean the entire 60-trillion member community of little neighborhoods and towns and states and countries which all together add up to the entire rich, complex experience of being You. And guess what?!

You, and you alone, are the Grand Poo-Bah in charge of this whole shebang!

Pretty cool, huh? You don't even have to run for office! You get to be the high potentate of You by simple virtue of being born—sort of like the royal family in England, only with better teeth! And you are elected for life!

But, here's the catch...you *still* have to worry about your polls. In the real world, what do communities of human beings do when their Leader treats them harshly or unfairly or even simply neglects their well-being. Well, at first, usually they do nothing. They just take it and suffer in silence. Humans can take a lot of neglect for a long time without speaking up. But eventually unease and dissent will crop up here and there, and before long people will express their dissatisfaction amongst themselves. If a Leader continues their ill-treatment of the populace for too long, finally the people will revolt!

The vast population of cells that have banded together to make up your body is no different. Your cells may well endure years and years of abuse and neglect without a single murmur of protest, but keep it up and sooner or later there's gonna be an uprising.

Instead of storming the Bastille, their revolt leads to lack of energy. Excess fat. Chronic sickness. Stroke. Heart attack. Type II diabetes. Good times, eh?!

Albert Einstein famously said we each have a

fundamental choice to make in life, 'Do we believe we exist in benevolent world, which is here to support and nurture us...or do we believe we exist in a malevolent world, which is out to get us and make us miserable and unhappy.'

All too many of us, Einstein noted, choose the latter. We go through life seeing the worst in the world, the worst in others and the worst in ourselves. In the same way, eventually each of us has to ask an even more fundamental question: Are we going to be a *malevolent* ruler of our empire of 60 trillion cells and continue zooming down the Fat Food superhighway. Or are we going to become a *benevolent* ruler and make a decision to slow down...and LIVE?!

As we'll discover in Secret #12, it's never too late to start being good to ourselves. It's never too late to lose the weight, restore our health and enjoy renewed energy in every cell of our body. And it's never too late to rediscover how to love our beautiful body the way we did when we little children.

There's a wonderful Chinese saying, "The best time to plant a tree is 20 years ago. The second best time to plant a tree is today!"

Lets decide to plant a tree today! Planting a tree means listening to the Audio Affirmations. Planting a tree means incorporating the 13 Progressions into our lifestyle, one at a time. Planting a tree means drawing a new line in the sand each day and reaffirming the belief that *we* are worth loving and our body is worth fighting for!

> *"To know oneself as a Body is more important, at this moment in history, than to read the words of all the wise men who have ever lived"*
> —Marco Vassi

SECRET #12:
"You Are Younger Than You Think"

I Can Guess Your Age!

What do you say we play a little guessing game?! Here's how it works: I'm gonna guess how old you are. Now you might be a little skeptical that I could possibly guess your correct age, since we quite possibly have not yet met in person.

But I should tell right you up front that I haven't missed yet!

Okay, you can help me guess by *thinking* of your age in your head right now. Just imagine your age vividly and mentally project it my way. Meanwhile, I'm going to put on Johnny Carson's old Karnak the Great headpiece, which will allow me to bend the space-time continuum and magically know your age. Nooooo, just kidding! I already know the answer...

You, good sir or madam, are about one year old! (By the way, Happy 1st Birthday!)

Your brain is already protesting this answer, right?! Because it thinks you are 18 years old or 81 or whatever number it *thinks*...and your brain is quite certain that it hasn't been one year old for a good long time now. See, your brain thinks of age in a strict *chronological* fashion — for which it uses reference points like the Date of Birth listed on your drivers license. What we're talking about here is your *biological* age — the equivalent of the rings on a tree that allow outside observers to know the tree's "true" age.

With all due respect to your local Department of Motor Vehicles, they really have no clue how old you are biologically. But just don't share any of what follows with the clerk at your neighborhood liquor store unless you want to get carded every time you walk in the door!

A Whole New You!

In an earlier chapter, we touched on how virtually every cell in our body gets replaced on a regular schedule. Well let's spend a few moments breaking down that schedule, because it will teach us something *critical* about our physical body that most of us were never, ever taught in school.

The cells on the surface of our tongues are totally replaced every *48 hours*—which explains why if we burn our tongue on hot soup or accidentally bite our tongue it pretty much stops hurting within a few hours and we usually forget all about it by the next day.

The cells lining our stomach rarely last more than *72 hours* before dying off and being replaced by an all-new starting line-up of stomach cells...which is a good thing because it's a grueling, acidic environment down there in our stomach!

Our entire epidermis—the "skin suit" that protects us from the big, bad outside world and is by far the largest organ in our Body, making up fully 15% of our total weight—undergoes a complete and total renewal every *14 days*!

Let's pause and consider the enormity of this never-ending construction job.

Every square inch of your skin contains about 20 blood vessels, 650 sweat glands and more than 1000 nerve endings...each and every one of which has to be reproduced perfectly in a mere 2 weeks—and then the process starts all over again, sort of like those guys who spend the entire year painting the Golden Gate Bridge and then the day after they finally finish they go back to the other end of the bridge and start all over again!

So 15% of us (almost the entire outside of us) is only 14 days old!

But an even larger percentage of us is made up of water. In fact, water makes up 60-70% of you. And every single drop of water in your Body is replaced every *30 days*!

So factoring together just our skin and body water replacement alone, some 75% or more of our body is between two and four weeks old! Your red blood cells have a consistent lifespan of *120 days*. During their brief tenure inside your magnificent body, they travel over 1000 miles through your intricate circulatory system...the walls of which also get replaced about every *3 months*!

Your liver is the master detoxifier of your Body. Well here's a lovely birthday present for you: You get a brand new liver about once a year—between 350-400 days!

If you're 43 years old, for example, then you've already had the benefit of some 40+ different livers! The rest of your organs and squishy bits also get replaced on similar schedules, ranging from 2 days from the high-use cells on your tongue to 9 months for your spleen.

Now your bones take a bit longer to get replaced, but over the span of 7-8 years, every single cell of every single bone in your entire body is replaced by all new ones!

How exactly does our body go about replacing our entire freaking skeleton without us collapsing to the ground inside a bone-less skin suit?!

Well, first, our body only replaces a minuscule amount of bone at a time—if it did a whole leg at once we would sort of fall on our face the next time we tried to walk!

And second, our body ingeniously employs two separate, specialized crews of worker cells. One crew goes in and literally dissolves the cells of a minute portion of one of our bones with an acid-like secretion...and then a second crew comes along and rebuilds the section with all new bone cells. Crazy the amazing things our incredible body can do, huh?!

Doing The Math

A quick recap...

Cells on top of tongue – 48 hours old

Lining of stomach – 72 hours old

Epidermis (top 3 layers of your skin) – 14 days old

The 60-70% of you made of water – 30 days old

Red blood cells – 120 days old

Liver – 350-400 days old

Bones – 6-8 old

When we average together the ages of all the cells that make up most of us, we come up with the approximate biological age of our physical body being just about 1 year old!

Which is a pretty staggering realization, if you think about it. I mean, not only are you the Emperor of a community of 60 trillion cells, but the average *age* of the inhabitants of your kingdom is merely one year old!

If you think about it, that really makes you more of a *babysitter* than a Grand Poo-Bah!

Ye Olde Kindergarten Teacher

Incredible as it may seem, our biological age is actually

considerably younger than one year old — it's our damn bones that skew the average so "high".

We completely replace a staggering 1% of our entire body each and every day.

That's an astounding, ongoing makeover job that deserves a reality show of its own! Of course, not every single cell gets replaced on this tight, 100-day schedule, but the fact remains that on average we're pretty much replacing our entire bodies every 100 days! In other words, YOU (and me, and everybody we know) have bodies closer to just *3 months old* rather than one year.

This begs the question, how then did we average out to being a whole one year old? Well, that's just the way math works!

Take a Kindergarten class with ten students, each of them 5 years old. The average age of the people in the classroom is: 5 years old. So far, so good — I got some mad arithmetic skillz, yo!! Now let's bring our teacher, Mrs. Jenkins, into the classroom. The old battle-axe just turned 60 yesterday. By introducing this one sexagenarian into the room we've skewed the numbers considerably. The average age of the people in the classroom is now: 10 years old!

This single 60 year-old teacher *doubled* the average age in the classroom. Similarly, at nearly 8 years of age our bones push our cells from an average age of a little over 3 months all the way to a full year old. Stupid bones! (JK, I love you, bones!)

By the way, there is *one* highly ironic exception to the rule that every single cell in our body gets replaced on a regular schedule.

We'll get to that exception in due course, don't you worry your pretty little head!

The 3 Tenets

The 3 tenets underlying the Low Carb Lifestyle are:

EAT FOOD

PLAY

LOVE

We've already explored each of these at length. And, on the face of it, this seems like a most reasonable way to treat the one-year old toddler that we are, wouldn't you say?!

After all, if you were a parent and had a little 12-month old baby, wouldn't you go to any length to provide your child healthy food to eat, a safe environment to play in and then bathe them in love day and night?!

So what's stopping us from treating our precious, year-old body with the same doting love and care that we'd give to any child?!

You're Only As Old As You *Think*

So many of us walk around telling ourselves sad stories such as, "Ohhhh, I'm 57 years-old and my body's all worn-out and tired and creaky!"

I'm here to tell you that's just another example of a *story* that's not useful...nor is it remotely true! Regardless of your chronological age, your biological body never ages beyond 1 year old on average. (And, again, *most* of you—over 85%, counting your water, epidermis and other squishy bits—is around 100 days old!)

What that means is that the eating and lifestyle progressions we discovered in Part One can make an almost immediate and dramatic effect on your actual, physical body as we implement them.

All those cells in your body, after all, are made up of

what you eat. When you change what you eat, you change what you're made of. By eating better, playing more and loving ourselves without reservation, instead of dragging around and complaining about our age all the time we can begin telling ourselves better stories such as…

"Yeeeehaw, I can remember celebrating 64 dang birthdays, but I've got the fresh, energetic, healthy body of one of them there lil' toddlers!" (For some reason, good news always sounds gooder with a Texas accent!)

The Fountain of Youth

Once you really *get* that your biological body averges only about 12 months old, then you'll undergo a paradigm shift where you also "get" that eating real food, playing frequently, and loving yourself, your tribe and the world around you is not only the best, but the only, way to treat your adorable, rosey-cheeked little body!

From time immemorial, we have scoured the planet in search of the celebrated Fountain of Youth. Drinking from this fountain was said to reverse aging and restore us to a younger, more youthful body. Well, we've now found it! And it was hidden in a place where so many of us were afraid to even look — *inside our own beautiful body!*

If you've spent any time studying the science of aging, then you already know that researchers have discovered there's no "built-in obsolescence" to the human body. There's nothing in nature that specifically states that our cells cannot keep on replacing themselves in perpetuity.

In other words, there are no scientific reasons why we cannot live to 100 or 120 or longer, if we desire, with complete health, energy and vitality. English longevity crusader Dr. Aubrey de Grey likes to say, "The first person who will reach 200 years or older is already alive today!"

The Exception That Proves The Rule

We come now to the "ironic" exception to the All Cells Constantly Replace Themselves Rule that I referred to earlier. It turns out that there is *one* community of cells that never gets replaced at all during our lifetime.

Although we can continually add new cells to this community, once they are created we're stuck with them for life, sort of like members of the U.S. Supreme Court! And these cells are found in our cerebral cortex, the gray stuff inside our skull. In other words, our brain! Which is indeed a supreme irony!

Our Mind — the very part of us that still *thinks* we're 35 or 65 years old — is pretty much the *only* part of us that actually is 35 or 65 years old! Unlike the rest of our body, none of the cells in our brain ever reproduce or replace themselves during our lifetime. We can (and do, every single day) add new neurons constantly, but we never replace existing ones.

The theory behind *why* we never replace brain cells is that if our mind went around "unhooking" synapses in order to replace them with new ones then our thoughts would become hopelessly jumbled.

To make up for this inability to replace existing cells, our brain is capable of astounding feats of plasticity — it continues to add synapses and connect them with already existing ones in increasingly complex ways throughout our entire life.

Mind vs. Body

Our brain cells are sort of like little celibate monks, separated from the real world behind the thick

monastery walls of our skull. And just as medieval monks despised physicality and sometimes even punished themselves (often in advance...I'm eying you St. Thomas Aquinas!) for any potential "sins of the flesh", our mind can similarly fall into an adversarial relationship with the body.

Well we've been working on repairing this relationship between mind and body throughout the entire book and we're about to go out with a bang! Although we certainly didn't think about it in these terms back when we were "actually" one year olds, in point of fact all of us were completely and obliviously in love with our bodies back then...and it's now time to return to that beautiful state of self-love and self-acceptance!

In the final chapter of the *Low Carb Revolution*, we're going to take the final, bold step in rebuilding the relationship between our beautiful minds and our beautiful bodies that will carry us into a remarkable future indeed!

> *"It is not time that ages the body, it is abuse that does."*
> —Herbert Shelton

SECRET #13:
"Losing Weight Is About Falling in Love"

Couples Counseling

Let's bring it home as we wind down the incredible journey we've gone on together here in the *Low Carb Revolution*. Over the last few years or even decades, as we became a little more unhealthy and overweight, it's likely we increasingly disconnected from our own bodies. At best we became apathetic about our physical bodies, at worst, downright angry and punishing.

If we want to continue restoring well-being and energy in our lives, we must continue working on our relationship with our bodies. No fitness plan or eating strategy in the world, mine included, will have any lasting benefit until we learn to love—really love and accept—our wonderful body.

I don't mean fall in love with our body once we finally get six-pack abs or buns of steel, but love and accept our body exactly the way it is right now!

How do we *show* our body how much we care?! It's no different than with any other relationship in our life—*by spending time together.*

I urge you to develop the habit of spending time with your body. Every single day. Not while listening to music and not while reading—those are simply additional opportunities to spend time with your mind, not your body. But rather just connecting with your body while walking around or dancing or playing.

The time has come for us to demonstrate a little love and respect for our body, no less than we share love and respect with someone we're in a serious relationship with...and relationships don't get any more serious than the one we have with our own body! We can all stand to communicate more with our body. That means, first and foremost, listening to it.

Instead of immediately dulling its messages with pills, potions and powders, we should listen to our body first and be open to what it's trying to communicate to us.

Whenever we get frustrated or feel that changes aren't happening fast enough, that the weight isn't dropping off at the exact rate our mind expects, we ought to remember who we're dealing with here—an amazing and precocious one-year old!

And the only way to communicate with a toddler is patiently and lovingly!

Commitment Time

The only way to accomplish anything in life is to commit to it. (This might seem pretty darn obvious, but you'd be surprised how many folks totally omit this step!) Commitment might start out as interest and then excitement, but for it to become real, for it to manifest itself in the world, our commitment ultimately has to explode into an enthusiastic, white-hot passion.

The passion of, say, a Revolution! If you're ready to draw a line in the sand, to finally stand up and fight for your beautiful body rather than against it, then you all you need to do is commit to it...and then follow through!

In the 13 Keys and the 13 Progressions of Part One of this book, you were exposed to radically new distinctions that have the potential to completely transform the way you view and treat your body.

You now finally understand the processes and mechanisms of how we actually gain weight and store fat, and you learned all the strategies and distinctions of better eating that will deliver you to the doorstep of your Ideal Body...if you will only commit to implementing them into your life!

This is an important stage of your life. Letting go of the belly fat that's been hiding beneath the surface for so long will always rate as one of the significant accomplishments of your life. It certainly is in mine!

The key to your success in continuing this journey is to make yourself the most important person in the world during this process.

You've given so much of yourself to those around you. It's now time to give back to yourself for a change. You've given so much love to the people in your life. Now you're need to give more love back to yourself. You've ignored (or worse) the "better half" of the most important relationship in your life...the permanent relationship you have with your beautiful body.

Well all that's gonna change from now on, isn't it?! As you implement to eating strategies of the *Low Carb Revolution* into your lifestyle, allow this to become one of the most magical periods of your entire life.

If you just give yourself *permission* to love yourself and treat yourself as the most important person in the world, then this can turn into a rebirth of your relationship with "you" as you lose weight, move your body more and more and finally "come home" to who you really are...allowing you Inner Self to emerge into the world, strong, powerful and ready to take charge!

Let your passion for loving and protecting your body build and percolate and infiltrate every cell. When you've got those internal fires stoked white hot — well, you're still just beginning! There's no *depth* to the love we can feel for our beautiful bodies! Returning to

458

our Ideal Body is one of the great achievements in life...not just because of the lost pounds but also because of what it represents. It's a direct reflection of how much we really, really, really, really, really--that's 5 really's!—love ourselves!

And above all, remember...*The Party Is In Your Body!*

> *"The two most important days of your life are the day you are born...and the day you find out why"*
> — Mark Twain

You 2.0

One of the greatest benefits to losing our belly fat and returning to our Ideal Weight is the go-go-go power it brings back into our lives.

A primary difference between the successful people we admire and those who are unable to get up out of their seats and join the Revolution can be traced to the increased energy and vitality of the former...and the sluggishness and energy-depleted procrastination-osity of the latter.

If you recall, I think of our personal *energy* as the power it takes to move our body through space. To accomplish our goals we sometimes need to take physical actions in the world.

Often that involves moving our body from Point A to Point B. If you're single and your goal is to find a romantic partner, but you don't have the energy to get dressed and get out of your house to go out dancing or go on dates, for example, it's going to be damn difficult to achieve your goal!

Vitality, on the other hand, I define as the power at our disposal when our body's not moving in any significant way.

In a real sense, vitality is our Inner Energy.

Vitality is the "idle" of our personality, the hum of activity and potential even when we're sitting still or engaged in conversation or thinking or writing. It's us firing on all cylinders on the inside, even while the outside remains calm and still.

To return to our earlier example, if you see a bear in the woods it takes energy to successfully run away from it. And that's all well and good, but if you subsequently want to write a blog post about escaping from the bear you're going to need a fair bit of vitality to sit down and write it. If anything, I consider vitality the more important and the harder to "muster up" of the two. Any fool can run around the block shouting at the top of his lungs. Only someone with sufficient vitality could sit down with a blank piece of paper in front of them and write a clever short-story worth reading about some fool running around the block shouting at the top of his lungs!

Together, our energy and our vitality lead to maximum goodness in our lives. As you incorporate the distinctions and strategies of Parts One and Two into your life you're going to have much more of both than you've probably experienced in years.

This gradual yet steady increase in your energy (what you can do in the physical world) and your vitality (how fast your circuits are firing on the inside) can be a little scary.

Because a bigger, more powerful engine under the hood also means that all those things you've always wanted to do in life, but ever had the energy or vitality to accomplish in the past, are now going to be possible for you.

That's why it's so important to write a Vision Letter, so you'll have a plan of attack, a map of your future to take you in the bold new directions you're now headed! (Hint-hint: If you skipped that step above, revisit the directions now and summon up the vitality to write your Vision Letter!)

> *"If you want to awaken all of humanity, then awaken all of yourself, if you want to eliminate the suffering in the world, then eliminate all that is dark and negative in yourself. Truly, the greatest gift you have to give is that of your own self-transformation."*
> —Lao Tzu

Let's Keep Falling In Love

Above all what we've learned together is that avoiding "beans", letting go of our belly fat and returning to our Ideal Body is fundamentally about falling in love with our beautiful bodies! The process of reconnecting with our body and becoming *aware* of it again can begin today…it can begin right now.

Just make a commitment right here and right now to yourself. *A commitment that you will remember to love yourself every day.*

Now I'm not talking about bubble baths or taking the time to read a trashy novel—although those are lovely and relaxing diversions, to be sure. No, I'm talking about loving and accepting and forgiving your body, just the way it is. Again…the party is in your body!

Rebuild that relationship and get used to connecting with your body and listening to it and working with it for a better you!

Imagine watching a young child on the playground. Running and climbing and swinging and fully inhabiting their body. They have no hang ups about their "body type", nor any awareness at all of a distinction between body, mind and spirit. There's no divide or barrier whatoever between Who They Are and What They Are (body).

Our goal, I strongly believe, is to return to that connection, to be in our bodies so completely that it's like we're children again—but with the experiences, resources and direction in life of an adult.

And that, my friends, is the path to happiness!

When you're ready, come back and share the discoveries you've made abour yourself, your body and the world with the rest of the class by writing a book of your own.

Learn exactly how to do that by visiting Amazon.com and picking up a copy of my 222-page book, *GET PUBLISHED NOW! The Step-by-Step Guide to Writing & Publishing Your First Book on Amazon Kindle!*

> *"I'm not the greatest; I'm the*
> *double greatest!"*
> —Muhammad Ali

I'm Gonna Miss You!

It's been my privilege and my pleasure to be your guide on the incredible journey we've just taken together. I'm seriously gonna miss you after we've shared this experience!

Remember to continue playing the Low Carb Lifestyle audio affirmations as often as possible in order to allow the positive messages about eating better, as well as playing and loving more, to sink into you on the deepest levels.

The audio affirmations will make this entire process so much smoother for you if you'll just take advantage of them.

And, if you haven't already, please tell others about my book, and let them know this is NOT a "diet book"...or at least it's nothing like any diet book they've ever read before!

I would also love it if you could make time in your busy schedule to write a short and sweet 5-star review on Amazon, because that will help influence others to take on themselves and go down the same road you've been going down.

I love you. Thank you for playing! And always remember: *YOU are worth loving...and your BODY is worth fighting for!*

"Be patient with yourself.
Self-growth is tender; it's holy ground.
There is no greater investment."
—Stephen Covey

The 13 Progressions of the Low Carb Revolution

1) *Eat as much as you want*
2) *Avoid Excess Sugars*
3) *Avoid Wheat Products*
4) *Drink Alcohol in Moderation*
5) *Avoid Processed Carbs*
6) *Avoid Drinking Sugars & Carbs*
7) *Avoid Natural Carbs*
8) *Mind your pH*
9) *Mix It Up*
10) *Cook It Yourself*
11) *Love*
12) *Create*
13) *Wake Up*

Printed in Great Britain
by Amazon.co.uk, Ltd.,
Marston Gate.